Along a Road of Acceptance

by

Jean Reid

2014

First published in 2014 by the author, Jean M Reid.

© Jean M Reid 2014

All rights reserved. No part of this publication may be reproduced, stored in a retrieval system, or transmitted in any form or by any means, electronic, mechanical, photocopying, recording or otherwise without the prior permission of the author, Jean M Reid.

jean@jeanreid.org.uk

ISBN 978-0-9929682-0-5

Printed in Great Britain by The Russell Press Limited, Russell House, Bulwell Lane, Basford, Nottingham NG6 0BT.

About the Author

Jean Reid was born in Chesterfield, Derbyshire in 1940. She attended Scarcliffe Primary School followed by two deaf schools—the Maud Maxfield School in Sheffield, Yorkshire and the Mary Hare Grammar School, a boarding school in Newbury, Berkshire. Jean has a dual sensory disability of hearing loss and sight loss—she is severely deaf and wears hearing aids and is registered as severely sight impaired. In 1959, Jean Reid found employment as a laboratory assistant at Robinson and Sons Ltd, a local firm that specializes in surgical dressings and boxes and about seven years later moved on to work in the Biochemistry Laboratory at the local hospital. She married Ronald Reid in 1971, they have two lovely daughters—Anthea and Sharon and five grandchildren—Jeanie, Joseph, Lauren, Ethan and Bryn.

Jean was a keen hockey player and played for Staveley Ladies in the Sheffield and District Ladies League and for Chesterfield Frolics, a mixed team that played friendlies and participated in hockey tournaments. Her hobbies are photography, family history, music, computers, walking in the countryside and she loves spending time with her family. Jean qualified as a guide dog owner and Ishka as a guide dog on 26th June 2012.

About the book

It was suggested that I should consider writing a booklet about my early years of coping with a dual sensory disability of hearing loss and sight loss. I have been hearing impaired since birth, thus I have grown up living with deafness, and the sight loss is due to Retinitis pigmentosa which developed during my teens. In my book, I have tried to describe my life and how I have moved from one identity to another as well as remaining essentially myself. My aim was to show that this has not all been a triumph or a tragedy but an ordinary happy life. Usher syndrome is the most common disease that affects both hearing and vision—it is a rare disease and there is no cure, but research is being done to find a much needed cure. People who have Usher syndrome face enormous daily challenges. So that my family know and understand more about how I coped in my earlier years I decided to write this booklet, but it has grown to more than just my early years and I feel that now I can share my experiences with a wider audience in the hope that it will make people more aware of this disease and help those who have Usher.

Acknowledgements

My thanks extend to several family members and friends for their encouragement, guidance and support. Special thanks to Ruth McLaughlin for planting that initial seed in my mind to write this book. I am also in debt to my granddaughter Jeanie Dowson—her computer skills are much better than mine! The advice that Susan Griffiths gave me about the printing process and self-publishing was invaluable and I appreciate Susan and Rosalyn Pursglove checking the book for errors—my thanks to both of you. A special thank you to my daughter, Sharon Reid for her help and encouragement, it was very much appreciated especially when I had 'writer's block' as she would come and sit with me whilst I talked and she typed. Thank you also to Julie and Lawrence for allowing me to use their photographs of Ishka; Julie and Lawrence were Ishka's puppy walkers.

Last but not the least, I would like to thank the late Mary Guest MBE for her help and encouragement in writing this book.

Also, thank you to FirstEditing.com for the editing service I received.

Jean M Reid 2014

In memory of my mum for her love and perseverance and to Ronald, my dear husband, for his love and moral support

Contents

Early Days 1

Maud Maxfield School 14

Mary Hare Grammar School 23

A Sudden Loss, Too Young 35

The Hearing World 47

At last, a diagnosis! 54

Ronald, my future husband 62

The Social Worker 71

The British Retinitis Pigmentosa Society 79

Communication 91

Ronald took Early Redundancy 96

Mobility 111

A change in circumstances 120

Charles Bonnet syndrome 131

Living with Ushers.. 135

Guide dogs Training 142

My Guide dog, Ishka 156

Appendix One: Ishka by Julie, the puppy walker............... 163

Appendix Two: Block Manual... 172

Appendix Three: Deaf/blind Manual Alphabet 174

Useful Addresses 179

ONE

My Early Years

I was born in Chesterfield, Derbyshire in 1940 to my mother Peggy Doreen and my father George Elliott. I was named Jean Mary. My father worked at Shirebrook Colliery as a fitter and, in his spare time, he was a keen local footballer and cricketer. Our family home was at Scarcliffe, a typical Derbyshire village situated about six miles from Mansfield and eight miles from Chesterfield, just two miles from the market town of Bolsover—many local people call the town 'Boza'.

To the south of Scarcliffe are Roseland and Langwith Woods, with Scarcliffe Park to the northeast. Most of the old charm still remains in the village, though new houses have been built to fit in with the old cottages and farms. The village is centred on the long main street, and includes a number of council houses at the top end of the village, with some new houses scattered about.

The Horse and Groom, a public house, lies at the top end of the village and is usually referred to as 'the top pub', while the Elm Tree—at the bottom end of the village—is appropriately named 'the bottom pub'. My great-grandfather, William Elliott, was the landlord of the Elm Tree for about eighteen years and then his son-in-law, Harold Cooper, took over.

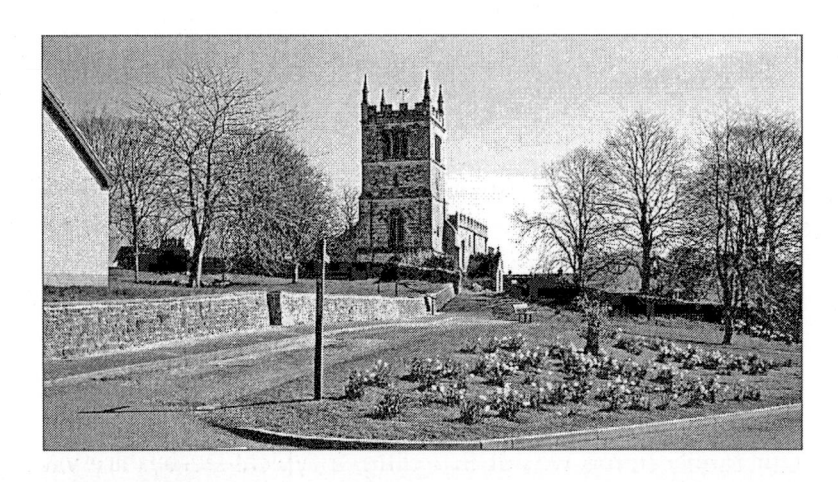

St Leonard's Church in Scarcliffe.

Towards the lower end of the village is the Norman parish church of St Leonard, where the alabaster tomb, dating back to the 13th Century, of Lady Constantia de Frecheville holding a child in her arms can be found.

As the story goes, Lady Constantia and the child were lost in the woodlands to the east of Scarcliffe, but the ringing of the curfew bell helped them find their way home to safety. The village also had a railway station, but it was closed on the 3rd December 1951. Until a few years ago, there was a Post Office and two shops that sold necessities, but for big shopping expeditions villagers tend to travel to neighbouring towns, such as Bolsover, Mansfield and Chesterfield.

The Second World War started on 3rd September 1939, and lasted until 1945. At the time I was much too young to know what was happening and how it was affecting the everyday life of people in this country or even our village. During the

Second World War, it became more difficult for our country to import products from other countries. Fruit, such as bananas, could no longer be imported, but small oranges were brought in and were saved for the children. Due to food shortages, the government introduced rationing, which enabled everyone to purchase the same amounts of food items at the same prices. We must not forget that food and essentials

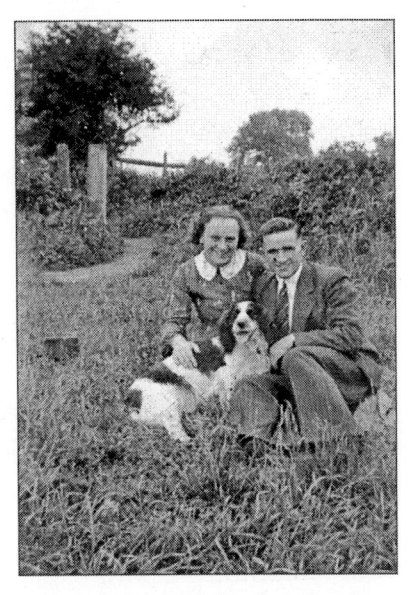

Mum, Dad and the family dog.

had to be supplied for our armed forces too. Everyone in the British Isles was given a ration book which had to be taken to the shops they had registered with to obtain rationed food items. Bacon, ham, butter and sugar were rationed first, followed by oil, margarine, cheese, marmalade, jam, syrup, treacle, eggs, sweets, chocolate and soap. The rationing programme turned out to be a big success, not only because of the fairness it implied, but also because it provided everyone with a healthy balanced diet. The government also came up with a policy called 'Dig for Victory' to encourage people to grow their own fruit and vegetables. Our milk came from a local farm—I can remember the milkman calling at our home with a churn and my mother giving him a jug to put the milk in. Rationing continued for many years after the war had ended. I can remember taking a ration book with me when

I went to the Mary Hare Grammar School in Newbury, Berkshire as late as 1952.

During the war, people had to cover their windows and doors with heavy black curtains to prevent any glimmer of light being seen by the enemy aircraft, especially during bombing raids. The street lights were turned off every night as well. I can remember seeing some pieces of heavy black cloth in a cupboard in my parents' bedroom after the war and, when I asked my mother what they were, she told me that they were curtains that covered the windows and doors at night during the war. Some evacuees came to live in Scarcliffe when the government recommended that the children should leave heavily-bombed London and move into the countryside. There was a girl from Croydon, London, who came to Scarcliffe during those years and became a very good friend of my Auntie Sis—they still keep in touch.

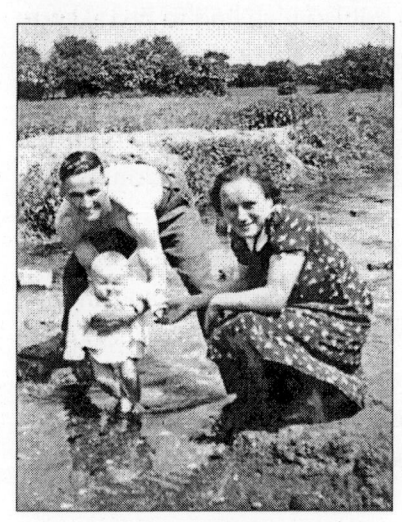

Mum, Dad and Jean.

One day when I was about five years old, news spread quickly through the village that there were some bananas for sale. Being such a rarity, this started a stampede to the village shop. I can remember standing in the long queue with my mother and cousin, Pat. I did not know what bananas were but seeing how everyone was so worked-up,

I too got carried away with the excitement. When I saw a banana for the first time in my life, I did not fancy it! Times were very hard during the war. There was not much money about and it was a tough time for everyone.

I cannot remember much about my father in the early years, as he was called up to serve the country during the Second World War, but I can recollect seeing two men in uniform calling at our home several times in an army truck, and one of them was my father. On one occasion, when I was about four years old, my father gave me a large box containing sweets that were wrapped individually in pretty, colourful paper. I did not know that they were sweets, as I most likely did not even know what sweets were at that time. My mother opened the box and I started to play with them, throwing them up into the air until they were scattered all over the floor. My mother picked one up and after unwrapping the sweet, gave it me to eat, but I spit it out because I was not used to the taste. I was told that the man who brought me this gift was my father, but that probably did not mean anything to me, as I was only a few years old and, given that my father was called up in 1941, I was not likely to have any memories of him.

I remember the times when my mother took me to the recreation ground where there were some swings and a large sand-pit that I enjoyed playing in. There was a football pitch as well, where the Scarcliffe football team played their games. Most of my father's brothers played for the team. In the 1940s we had much greater freedom than the children have to-day and I have some very happy memories that I would like to share with you. The local children could roam at will and stay outdoors for hours without any supervision or restrictions on their play. When I was old enough, I was allowed to join them.

There was also a much stronger sense of community back then as, if we were thirsty, we could knock on anyone's door and ask for a cup of water. If I fell down and grazed my knee, my mother would wipe it clean and put some yellow stingy iodine on it. I hated the stuff, though not enough it would seem, to stop me from falling over again! On fine days, especially on Sundays, many families would take jam sandwiches and a bottle of water and spend the entire day at the brook, where the neighbourhood children could play all day, paddling, building dams, or even climbing trees—we had lots of fun. The adults and older children played football or cricket.

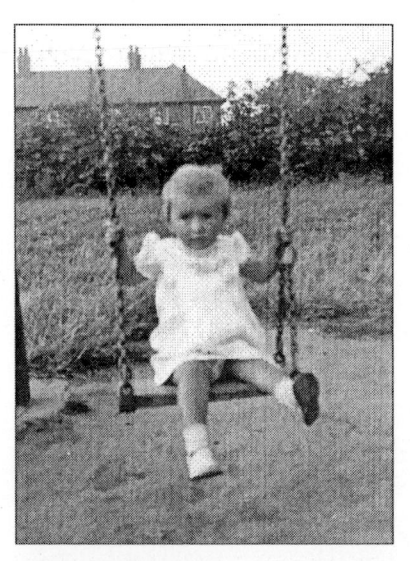

Jean on a swing.

We had skipping ropes, roller skates, marbles, whip and top, all of which provided lots of fun. Sometimes we would have a long rope that we used as a skipping rope. Everyone could join in, but we first had to persuade adults to turn the rope for us. We played some skipping games when some of my friends would sing songs and we would have to follow the instructions. You probably guessed correctly that I was not very good at this, but I still had lots of fun, as I would usually be skipping for much longer than some of the other children did—I did not know the songs and never knew when I had to skip in or jump out!

I was not one for playing with a pram and dolls, preferring to play football, cricket, tig, or hide-and-seek instead. For me, outdoor activities were much more fun—I enjoyed playing hopscotch, leapfrog, and conkers, and playing 'Cowboys and Indians' with the other children. I was proud to be able to wear a marvellous Indian outfit that my mother made me for a fancy dress competition at a carnival held at the village. I did not win, but I was delighted with it and wore it during our games. We did not have electronic devices, such as video games, computers, and transformers, which children seem to enjoy nowadays.

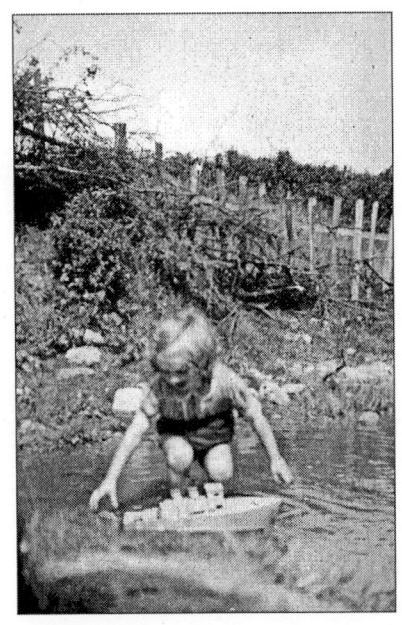

Jean paddling down at the brook.

At harvest time, I enjoyed riding on the tractor with Uncle Harold, who helped out at the farm—he would let me hold the steering wheel with him, which was so exciting! First, the corn was cut, and then farm workers would follow, gathering the corn up and tying it into sheaves. Finally, the sheaves would be stacked up into stocks. The men with the pitchforks would load

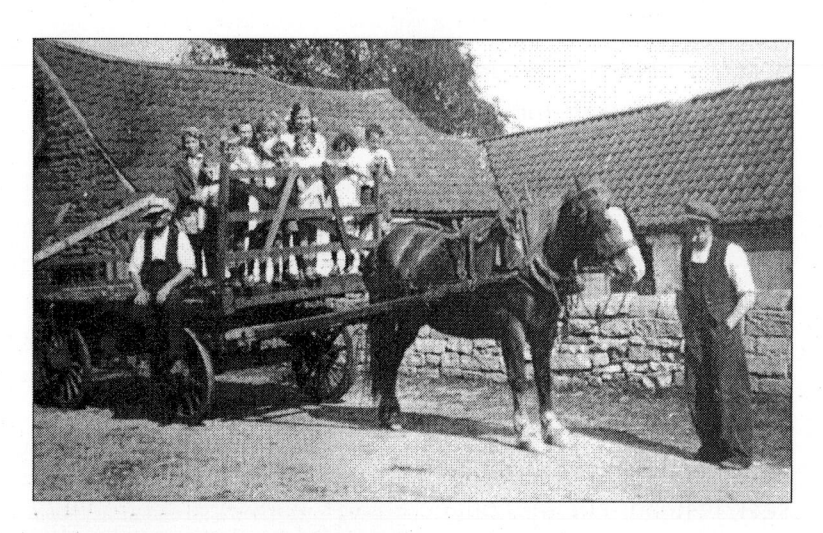

The ride back to the fields.

up the carts by throwing the sheaves up onto the carts where another farm worker would stack them up neatly before they were taken back to the farm. On its way back to the fields, the cart would be loaded up with the village children, who would enjoy the ride—my mother took the photo above.

My mother did a lot of baking and, being an accomplished dressmaker, she made most of our clothes. She also helped other people who wanted alterations done to their clothes; nothing was too much trouble for her. I can remember a red dress with little white flowers that my mother made for me; it was lovely and was my best dress that I would wear on special occasions. In those days we always had a best dress.

My mother was a member of the Women's Institute (WI), an organisation that helped to care for evacuees during the Second World War. Although devoted to this cause, the Institute is better known for their contribution to growing and preserving foods.

My mother was hard working and had a strict sense of values. Even though corporal punishment was acceptable in those days, she preferred other forms of disciplining. So, when I was naughty, my mother would send me to my bedroom for a while. As there were no books or toys in the bedroom, all I could do was look out of the bedroom window and watch my friends playing and having a good time. I had to stay in the bedroom until my mother called me downstairs again. I can remember one such occasion when, after some time, I got bored of just sitting in my bedroom and decided that I had been punished for long enough. I went downstairs and told my mother that, if she said that she was sorry, I would go out to play. Much to my surprise, for some reason she did not agree! Auntie Ruth always enjoyed telling people this story, so I was unlikely to ever forget it. I got into trouble many times for running out on to the road without looking to see if there were any cars coming. I had some lucky escapes!

Auntie Ruth and Uncle Harold lived on the edge of the village. They had a large orchard full of apple and plum trees, where my uncle also kept fowls. I loved helping to feed the fowls and collect the warm eggs, but there was one thing that I did not like—a rather vicious cockerel. I had to hide behind my uncle's back, as he walked slowly through the orchard, carrying a stick for protection. In one part of the garden, my uncle grew raspberries, blackcurrants and gooseberries as well as many types of flowers. I enjoyed picking the fruit and helping Auntie Ruth to pack the apples in boxes ready to store in the box-room. There was always some homemade jam and chutney in her large pantry and I enjoyed the delicious jam sandwiches that she made for me. When I was older Auntie Ruth showed me how to make homemade jam.

The highlight of the week was when Mr Johnson came to Scarcliffe with his horse and cart, selling fruit and vegetables. I really looked forward to his visits. The other children would run to the houses shouting, letting the neighbours know that he was there, but I preferred to stay behind, as I was always chosen to ride in front of the cart and hold the heavy leather reins. The horse pulling the cart was called Trigger and I liked him very much. We would go to every house in the village and would usually be treated to an apple for our efforts.

The gas lamps that were used as street lighting at the time did not give off much light. There was one halfway down East Street that became a sort of a meeting place for the children who lived nearby. We knew everyone who lived in the street, actually we knew everyone that lived in the village! In the evenings, we liked to play Hide and Seek, as the neighbours did not seem to mind us hiding in their gardens. We also played marbles until some parents, usually Mrs Heath, who lived nearby, started shouting out that it was time for us all to go home. She used to scare the daylights out of us by telling us that, if we did not hurry, the bogeyman would come and get us! At about this time, my Uncle Jack would be walking up the street on his way to the top pub and would join in by shouting out that the bogeyman was, indeed, coming—that did scare me and made me run home fast! When I went to bed, I would look in my drawers, inside the wardrobe and un-

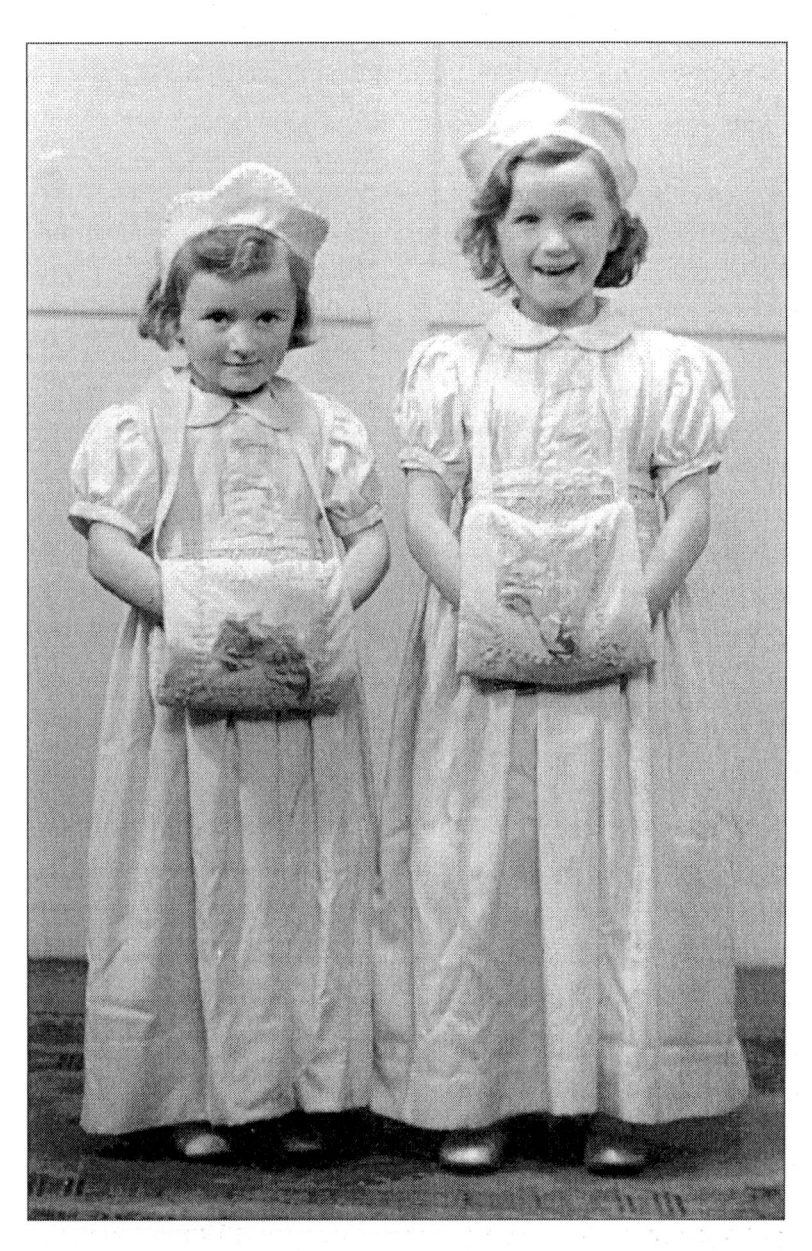

Bridesmaids Jean and her cousin Pat.

der the bed to see if the bogeyman was there before getting into bed. Of course, there was no such thing as a bogeyman.

I enjoyed going roller-skating with my friends down Fox Hill—a steep hill at the bottom end of the village. There were not many cars in those days and there was no bus service through the village, so the only things that we had to watch out for were horse-drawn carts and tractors. If someone was going down the hill on their skates and saw a tractor, they would call out 'Tractor' as loudly as they could and everyone would drop off their skates, or they would most likely end up in the hedge bottom! I was always the last one to respond and usually ended up in the hedge bottom. My mother would get very annoyed with me when she found out because I was not allowed to go roller-skating down Fox Hill.

During the winter months, when the snow came, we would go tobogganing down Lockey Hill, a steep hill just outside the village. One family owned a large red sledge, which would go very fast down the hill. If they were very lucky, or rather unlucky, they would end up in the stream at the bottom of the hill. Whenever they sledged down the hill, people would cheer if they got near to the stream without falling in. Some villagers would build snowmen while others would take part in snowball fights. You can be sure that everyone had a great time on the snowy hill. We would return home wet and cold and my mother would make us all a hot cocoa and some toast. We would enjoy the treats, as we sat in front of the warm coal fire.

Although I was very young at the time, I can still remember the heavy snowfalls of 1947 that disrupted the village as well as the entire country. There was so much snow and it was very deep. The village was cut off and we were running out of food. In those days, as we did not have fridges or freezers, all the food was kept in the cold pantry and dairy products and perishables such as meat and cheese were kept in a meat-safe placed on the cold stone. Now, you may wonder what a meat-safe is—I will tell you. It was a three-sided mesh cupboard that protected meat and cheese from flies and other insects. Eventually, a message was sent to the village from a farm in Palterton, situated about a mile away from the village. They had some bags of potatoes and, although they were happy to let anyone that wanted some to have them, they would not be able to deliver them. Many men from the village set out to the farm with their sledge to fetch some bags of potatoes. As they were gone for a long time, some families started getting a bit worried and volunteers went out to help to bring the much-needed bags of potatoes home. My father and his brothers finally got home cold, wet and very weary. When the snow started to melt, the water came down from the fields via Fox Hill to the bottom of the village and down the main street. As a result, the lower part of Scarcliffe village was flooded for days.

TWO

Maud Maxfield School

When I was five, I attended Scarcliffe Primary School, which was a small school, situated at the bottom end of the village, near the church. As I did not make good progress with my school work, I was considered a backward child—what would today be viewed as a person with learning difficulties. However, one day, a new headmistress named Mrs Groves arrived at the school. I can still remember Mrs Groves sitting in the classroom, observing our class at work, but I did not realise that she was actually assessing me. Observing me in class, she must have noticed that I did not respond to any loud noises made in the classroom and that I did not always know when the teacher was talking and that I seemed to daydream a lot which suggested that I was hearing-impaired.

Following a discussion with my mother, it was agreed that I should see the school doctor, who put me in a corner facing the wall and told me to say 'yes' whenever I heard his voice, which is what I did. He then declared that I was not suffering from hearing loss. Later that day, my mother asked me if I could really hear what the doctor was saying. I explained that I could hear his voice, but I did not know what he was saying.

Thankfully, my mother never gave up, as she was aware that there was something not quite right with her daughter. It must have been an anxious time for her, being on her own while my father was still away. I was about eight when it was confirmed that I was partially deaf and thus became a pupil at the Maud Maxfield School for the deaf in Sheffield, Yorkshire.

Travelling every day to school was a long tedious journey that started on the 7.50a.m. service bus and lasted for about one and a quarter hours. The same journey was repeated after school. At first, my mother travelled with me to Sheffield and then returned later to collect me at the end of the school day. Looking back, it must have been very tiring for her and must surely have been a big drain on the family income. However, unknown to my father, Uncle Ken, my mother's brother, helped out with the travelling expenses. I did not know at the time that my grandma and Uncle Ken did not approve of my father and refused to attend my parents' wedding—my mother married my father as soon as she was twenty-one. My grandma and Uncle Ken were never really on speaking terms with my father after that.

Eventually, it was suggested that I travel to Sheffield on my own. There were some other children on the public transport attending school in Sheffield. Even though we were attending different schools, over time, I had become friendly with them. Auntie Mary, my father's sister, was a conductor on the East Midland Bus Service and asked her colleagues to keep an eye on me. When I got on the bus in the mornings, the conductors would say, 'Come on Jean, let's have you on'. I always went on the top deck to the front of the double-decker bus.

At this school, I learned how to lip-read and was given some speech training, as it was called in those days. I can remember sitting in front of a large oval mirror with the teacher sitting beside me, learning how to pronounce individual letter sounds, syllables and, finally complete words. I started with the following consonants; m, n, b, f and p. My teacher used 'props' such as a feather, a strip of paper and a balloon to help me to pronounce consonants—she used a feather to illustrate the 'f' letter. As she pronounced the letter 'f', she would breathe out onto the feather that she was holding in front of her mouth. She put my hand on her throat to feel the vibrations of her voice as she spoke—I could ascertain differences in vibration for different sounds. There are some letter sounds that vibrate in the nose such as 'm' and 'n'. When the teacher showed me how to pronounce 'n', she would put her forefinger on the side of her nose and pronounce 'n' then she would put my forefinger on her nose so that I could feel the vibration—it would make me laugh. I would then try and pronounce 'n' with my forefinger on the side of my nose. I had to practise words containing 's', 'sh', 'st' and 'ch'—they were the ones I had the most difficulty in pronouncing.

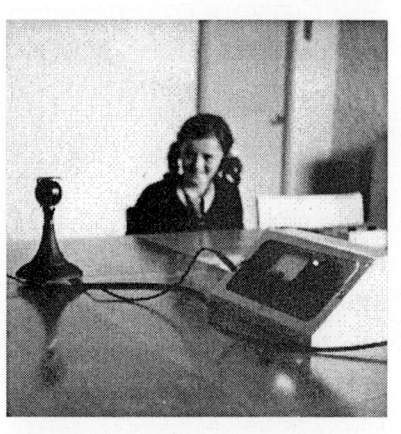

Speech training at the new school.

Lip-reading is a communication skill based on watching the lips of the person you are talking to—a method that I used along with the bulky, heavy and uncomfortable hearing aid that I had to wear, so much different to the digital hearing aids that I wear today.

The classrooms were so much smaller then, with about nine pupils, each at his own desk. After about three weeks, I was moved up to the next class, this move would have pleased my parents as it showed that I was making some good progress. All the teachers spoke slowly and clearly, which enabled me to hear and understand what they were saying. There was certainly no cheating, which was common at Scarcliffe Primary School, when I would copy off my friends for I did not understand what I had been told to do, as my deafness prevented me from following the lessons.

Most of the children at the school used the sign language and it was certainly not surprising that I initially found it very strange watching them waving their hands about and making funny facial expressions and noises. I did not know then that these facial expressions were part of the sign language. I settled down quickly at this school and was really happy there in that environment. I was never taught to use the sign language properly by the other children, though now I wish that I had been. It was not long before the school moved to some new premises on Ringinglow Road, which meant yet another bus ride for me.

On the first day of attending school in the new location, one of the teachers met my mother and me at the bus station in Pond Street, and together we caught the bus to the new school. This certainly made it a long journey for me—however,

I felt much safer having some adult company with me on my first day at the new school, not to mention the surprise I got when, before going to join my classmates, I was told to report to the kitchen where I was given a hot drink of cocoa and some biscuits—from then on, I had to report to the school kitchen every morning before going into class.

I really enjoyed my time at the Maud Maxfield School, as we had plenty of opportunities to explore new things and enjoy experiences we would not have had otherwise. One of my fondest memories was that I took part in two plays—*Pied Piper of Hamelin* and *Sleeping Beauty*. In the first play, *Pied Piper,* the main character, was a rat-catcher hired to lure the rats away. When the town refused to pay for his services, Pied Piper retaliated by using his magic pipe on the children, leading them to their demise. I played the part of Hans, one of the children and loved the green tunic and brown stockings that I wore as a part of my role. In the other play, *Sleeping Beauty*—the story of a beautiful princess who was destined by a curse to prick her finger on a spindle of a spinning wheel and become Sleeping Beauty—I played the part of a fairy, which I also loved, as I was thankfully not the horrible one, but a nice one! The school also arranged a day-trip to Lincoln that I enjoyed—especially the visit to the cathedral.

Despite every effort made by the school staff to make us feel comfortable with our disabilities, looking back, there has always been a certain stigma surrounding deaf people. The issue is probably not as pronounced today, but in the old days we were treated differently from others. If someone was deaf, out of sheer ignorance, people tended to assume that they were slow or backward. Clearly, this is rarely the case, as the only problem most deaf people have is that they cannot hear and, as a result, cannot always understand speech. If people wear glasses, there is no stigma attached to them, as there is with hearing aids that most deaf people wear, to help amplify the sounds coming to their ear. In addition, even though many deaf people sign instead of using their voice, most deaf people can pronounce words, albeit differently from those with good hearing. You must understand that, if someone is unable to hear his own voice, it is likely that his voice will sound funny to you. Still, what I cannot understand is why so many people, when in the presence of a deaf person, start to speak louder or even shout. It makes me wonder why they believe that if they do this, the deaf person will be able to hear them better. Not only is this humiliating, but, as the speaker's voice becomes distorted, shouting also makes it more difficult for the deaf person to recognise some of the words used. This has happened to me many times, especially when I was a little girl. There was one lady who lived in my village whom I would dread seeing, who would come very near to me and practically shout down my ear, making me cringe! How she did not burst my eardrums, I will never know.

Although most people know this already, I still think that it is worth explaining that, when talking to a deaf person, all you have to do is make certain that you are facing them. It is important to talk clearly, but it is not necessary to shout. Other things to consider when talking to a deaf person are to make sure that the light is falling on your face and, if you are indoors, make sure that you are not sitting or standing in front of a window. If you are, the deaf person may not be able to see your face and will be unable to lip-read you. Although many people are still uncomfortable with directly addressing someone's disability, do not be embarrassed if the deaf person asks you to repeat what you have just said, as they would most likely not have understood everything in the first place. It is possible to communicate with deaf people even without the use of sign language. Still, there are some deaf people who prefer not to use their voice, opting instead to use sign language. Many deaf people do use their voice and it may take some getting used to their pronunciations.

For a long time, I had no idea who Miss E Maud Maxfield was; hence, I decided to do some research. Here is a brief summary of my findings regarding Miss Maxfield and the school. East Hill House was the home of Alderman John Wycliffe Wilson and his wife, Ruth. John Wycliffe Wilson had a long and distinguished career, becoming a member of Sheffield City Council in 1890 and Lord Mayor during 1902–1903. His wife, Ruth, was also actively involved in Nether Chapel and education, becoming the first woman to be appointed to the Sheffield Schools Board, where she served for nine years. They were friends and colleagues of Miss Maxfield, who was also a member of Nether Chapel and had a keen interest in education. From 1894, Miss Maxfield was also a member of the Sheffield Education Committee, her special interests being the care of mentally and physically defective children as well as children who were deaf and blind.

Following the death of John Wycliffe Wilson in 1921, his son, Talbot Wilson, sold East Hill House to the Sheffield Education Committee for use as a day school for deaf children. Until then, deaf children from Sheffield attended Deaf Institutions as boarders in Doncaster, Manchester, and Derby. However, as it was decided that deaf children should attend a school in Sheffield, where they lived, East Hill House was an ideal solution, being a large house surrounded by gardens, playing fields and with easy reach of the town centre.

Miss Maud Maxfield was involved with arranging all this and the schools founded at East Hill were named after her. East Hill, which became the Maud Maxfield School for the Deaf, opened in 1922. There was also a school for the partially sighted, the Myope School, which opened in 1923 and was housed in three ex-army huts placed near the entrance gates. Miss Maud Maxfield always took an active interest in both schools and was a frequent visitor until she died in February 1940. The Maud Maxfield School closed in 1981.

In 1952, it was suggested by the headmistress, Miss B Elliott that I should take the entrance examination for the Mary Hare Grammar School, a school for the deaf in Newbury, Berkshire which would mean that I would become a boarder, should I pass the entrance exams. My mother was keen because she knew that it would open up more opportunities for me, but some family members were opposed to the idea, saying that I would be better off staying at home with the family. There were many arguments, and it must have been very distressing for my mother, but my father made it known that he would support any decision that my mother made. I took the entrance examination on 6th February 1952—the day that King George VI died and Princess Elizabeth became Queen at the age of twenty-five.

My mother was thrilled to bits when she heard that I had passed the entrance examination for the Mary Hare Grammar School—a residential school for the deaf in Newbury, Berkshire. Still, as all mothers, she must also have been concerned, wondering if I would settle at this new school, so far away from home. Although I was happy at the Maud Maxfield School and had some lovely friends there, I was really looking forward to going to the Mary Hare Grammar School.

THREE

Mary Hare Grammar School

I can remember vividly the day when I walked through the main oak door of Arlington Manor as a first year pupil. As I found myself in a large oak-panelled hall, I noticed a grand piano on the left and a magnificent wooden staircase on the right. Although the staircase dominated the hall, my attention was drawn to the half-portrait of a lady in green before me. I later learned that this was a painting of Miss Mary Hare, the lady responsible for giving deaf children the chance to have the best education they could possibly have. Green was apparently Miss Hare's favourite colour, which was why the school uniform was green. I still find it hard to believe that I had music lessons, when I was given the opportunity to play on the grand piano in the hall.

The Mary Hare Grammar School was founded on 1st January 1946 at Dene Hollow in Burgess Hill, Sussex and opened on 30th April 1946 with forty seven pupils as its first boarders. In 1949, the school moved to Arlington Manor, a Georgian mansion standing in an estate of woodland and parkland and situated about three miles north of Newbury. The school drive was lined with rhododendron bushes, and in spring there was always a wonderful display of daffodils in front of the manor house. Positioned among the evergreen trees, the manor always looked splendid, especially owing to its magnificent surroundings. The school was officially opened by

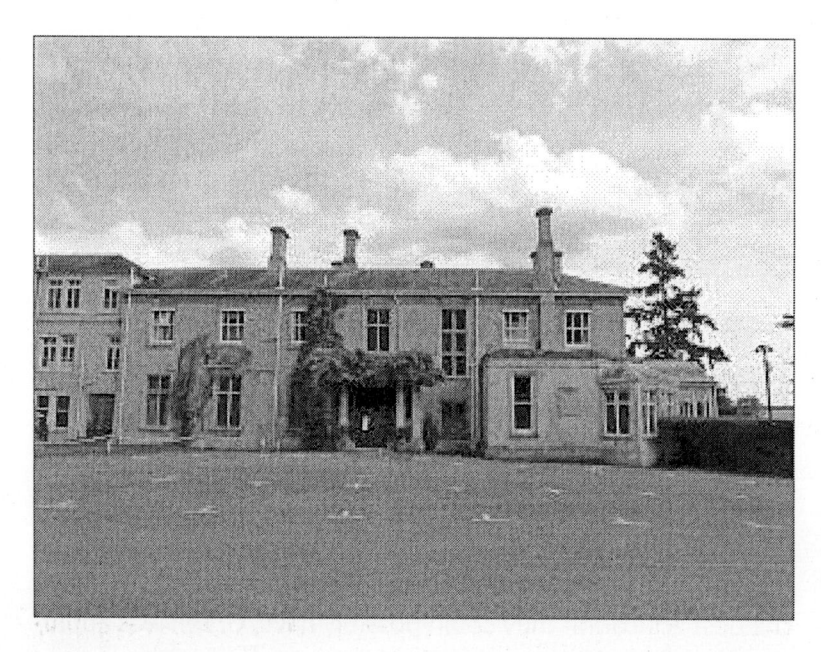

Arlington Manor 2012

Princess Margaret on 19th July 1950—this was, obviously, a memorable occasion for the Mary Hare Grammar School.

Mary Adelaide Hare (1865–1945) believed that deaf and mute children did not need protecting in institutions and that they should be allowed to have an education. Miss Hare began her career as a teacher of the deaf in 1883 by establishing a small school in London. Later, the school moved to West Sussex, where it became known as the Dene Hollow Oral School for the Deaf. Miss Hare was determined to show the hearing world that deaf children were capable of academic success. Today, the Mary Hare organisation still follows Miss Hare's principles, determined to give deaf children the opportunity for academic success.

I was placed in Helen Keller dormitory, named after the well-known American deaf/blind graduate, authoress and legend and one of the main characters in the film *The Miracle Worker*, which was basically about Ann Sullivan, Helen Keller's teacher. All the dormitories were named in honour of pioneers in the teaching of deaf children, such as Alexander Graham Bell, St John of Beverley, Thomas Arnold, and Thomas Braidwood. There were four houses: Arnold (red), Beverley (yellow), Braidwood (blue), and Mary Hare (green)—I was placed in Braidwood House.

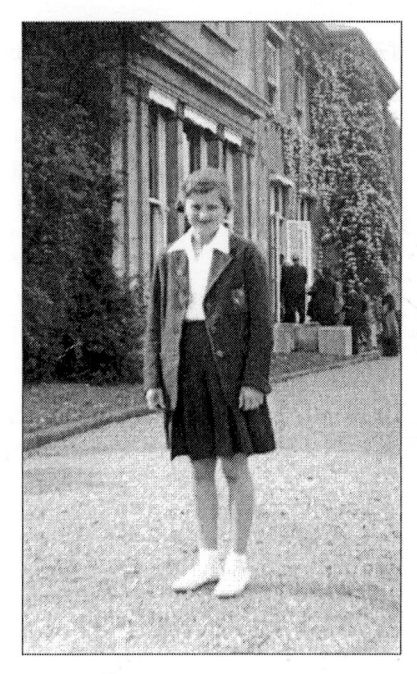

Jean Elliott, Sports Day 1953

There were seven or eight beds in Helen Keller dormitory. The walls were bare as the school rules did not allow us to put posters or pictures on the walls. Bedtime rules were strict and we were supposed to be in our beds before set times—then the lights were switched off by the girls' matron and woe betide anyone who was not in bed by then. We had to rise at 7.00a.m., wash, dress and strip the bed before going down to the dining room for breakfast. After breakfast, we would return to our dormitories, make our beds and make sure that we left our dormitories tidy before collecting our mail.

The school day started at 9.00a.m. with assembly in the hall and finished at 4.00p.m. After tea, served at about 4.30p.m., we would return to our classrooms to do our homework under the supervision of a school prefect. After supper, served at about 7.00p.m., most of the pupils would go into the General Purpose Room to play chess, table-tennis, chat to friends or read a newspaper or library book. We had an old gramophone in the General Purpose Room, but only one record that we played often—no wonder the headmaster got fed up of hearing it, as the record was *Cry* by Johnny Ray and obviously we would have the volume up high.

On Saturday mornings, the boys would wear their dungarees and do some work in the school grounds while the girls would do their mending. The teacher on duty would have a list of the girls who had some mending to do, which was compiled when the clothes returned back from the laundry and were checked for any holes or flaws. All the girls had to report to the domestic science room to do their mending. This could involve sewing buttons on our blouses, putting some new elastic in our green school pants, or darning a hole in our stockings. Once the mending has been done, it was checked by the teacher on duty. If she considered the work to be satisfactory, some other work would be found for us to do, otherwise the mending would have to be done again.

When some girls had finished their mending, they would be sent to help out in the kitchen, peeling apples or something similar. Some others, including me, would take our time doing the mending, making it last all morning if possible, knowing that, once enough girls had gone to help in the kitchen, more enjoyable jobs would be found for us. Unfortunately for us, the prefects must have realised what was going on, as later they started a rota, so that all the girls had to take turns doing some work in the kitchen.

I loved games—the girls played netball and hockey during the winter and in the summer it was rounders, tennis, and athletics. The boys played football in the winter and cricket, tennis and athletics during the summer. Matches were played against local schools. When the boys practised their cricket skills in the nets, I would join them, as I loved playing cricket. My father was a local cricketer and my uncle, Charles Elliott, played for Derbyshire County Cricket 1st XI and went on to become a top class test umpire. As for my great uncle Harry Elliott, he was Derbyshire and England wicket keeper; you can see why I loved cricket.

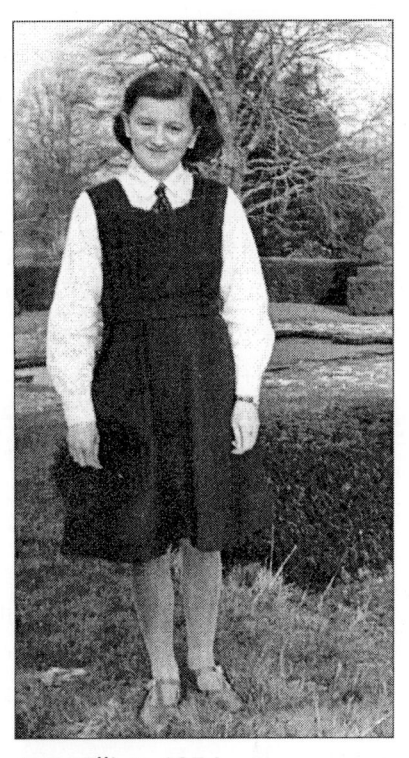

Jean Elliott 1954

There were also some clubs that we could join, such as Rabbit Club, Badminton Club, Pig Club, and Girl Guides. On Sunday mornings, we went to church, wrote letters to our parents, read newspapers or magazines, and after lunch, followed by a siesta, we would go out for a walk on Snelsmore common or to Donnington Castle, a ruined medieval castle, situated in Donnington, a small village just north of Newbury. After lunch one Sunday afternoon, our names were called out and the headmaster took a group of us out in the school bus into the countryside. He gave us a map and after pointing out where we were, left us to find our way back to school. We all enjoyed it very much and this was when I became interested in map reading. On another occasion, about six of us were treated to a boat trip on the River Thames with the headmaster and his wife—I believed the boat belonged to the headmaster.

In 1953, the BBC made a film about the school, featuring a scene with our class playing with the rabbits. Most of the juniors were members of the Rabbit Club—we took it in turns to feed the rabbits and clean the rabbit huts out. After being told when the film would be broadcast, I wrote a letter to my mother, asking her to watch the television on a certain day at a certain time, I did not want to tell my mother why, as I wanted it to be a surprise for her. As it happened, on the day, my cousin Pat was there and she switched the television off, telling my mother that it was a programme for deaf children! So, my mother never did see that film, which is a shame as there was a lovely shot of me holding a rabbit.

We were not allowed to have pillow fights but we did have one and got caught! Mind you, we had a great time jumping on the beds and hitting each other with our pillows even though the punishment was to clean all the girls' wellingtons and plimsolls. A group of girls got caught having a midnight

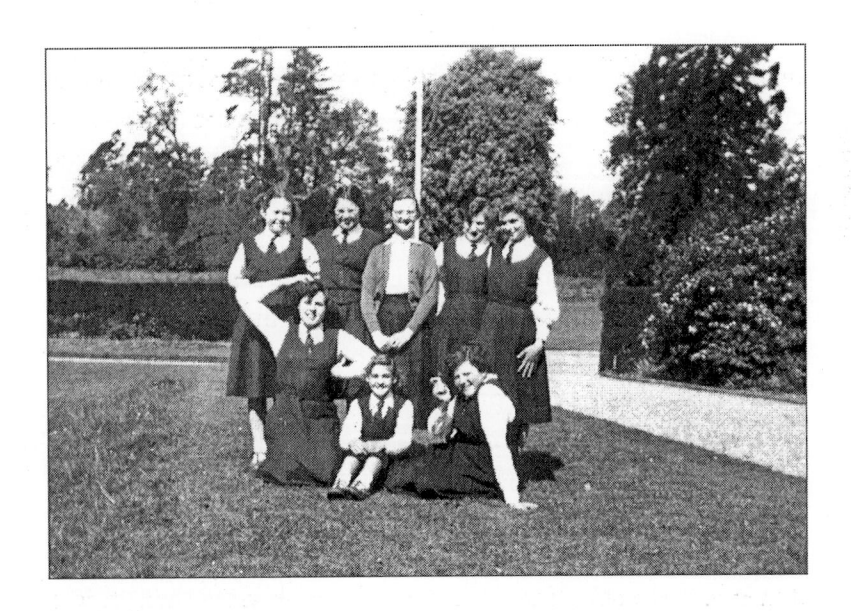

Happy school days.

feast in the bathroom, of all places! That was rather risky, as the bathroom was only a few metres from the girls' matron's room. They were bettered by a group of junior girls who hid the food and had the midnight feast in the prefects' common room. The leader of this group had the cheek to let me know when they had had the feast. I was the Senior Prefect and Head Girl at the time and the one who had to organise a search party to find the food—we searched all over the place but without success.

On my last day at the school, the group of girls who had the midnight feast came to my bedroom, poured some cold water over my face while I was asleep and then all jumped on to my bed. It was obviously a single bed and I still don't know how it survived! I asked the girls where they had their midnight feast and they told me that they had it in the prefects' common room. If the prefects had found the food, they could have had a feast—albeit not at midnight. I wondered what the girls would have thought had they found all the food missing when they went down to the prefects' common room for their midnight feast! Later, as I pondered on this hilarious turn of events, I was not so sure about the prefects having a feast, given that the girls hid their food behind the box containing the lost property and goodness knows what had been in there!

The Mary Hare Grammar school is an oral school and this brings me to the dreaded speech competition. At this school it was compulsory for all pupils to speak with their voices and not use the sign language—most pupils did sign to their friends when they thought that there were no teachers in the vicinity. All the teachers carried a little book and, if they saw any of the pupils signing or communicating without relying solely on their voice, their name would go in the book, hence losing a point. The House with the most points remaining at the end of the school term would win the Speech Trophy.

During my time there, new buildings continued to be added to the school, including classrooms, school hall, and gym. However, since I left the school in 1959, so much more has been added that I am certain that I would not recognise the school now. Some new school buildings were opened on the 24th October 1958 at the Eleventh Annual Speech Day. The Guest of Honour was Lord Kilmaine and I remember this well as I was the Senior Prefect and Head Girl and had to give the Vote of Thanks to our guests.

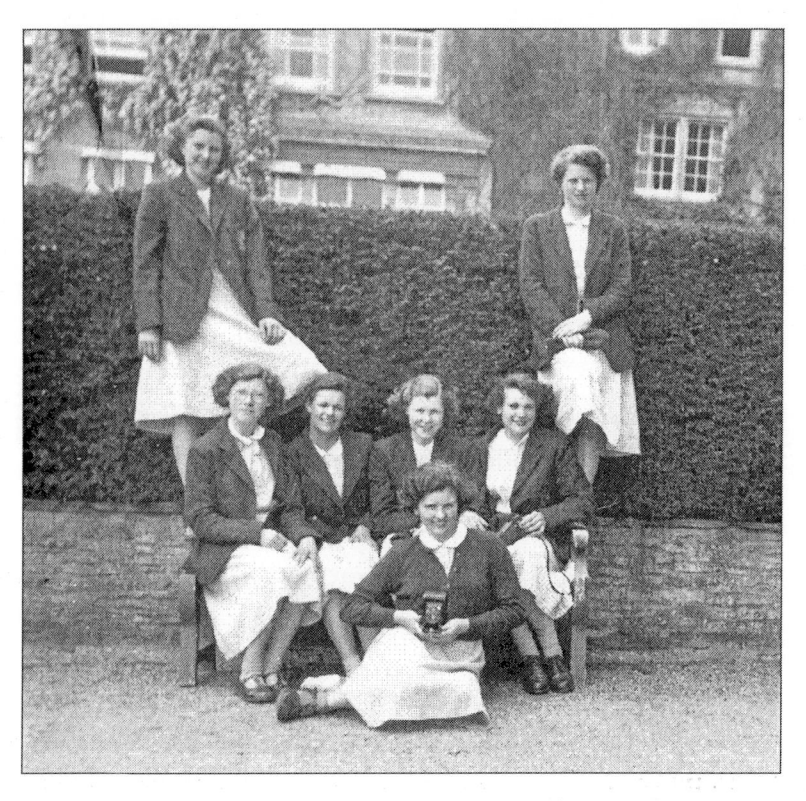

Friends together.

We were allowed to have our cycles at school but had to obtain the Cycling Proficiency Badge before being allowed to cycle to church or Newbury. The school had a tuck shop that opened at certain times every day, when we could buy sweets, crisps, chocolates, and small bottles of pop. When I started at the Mary Hare Grammar School, I still had a ration book, which limited the amount of sweets I could buy. When I was a senior pupil, I helped out at the Tuck Shop. We had a school bank, where we could deposit our pocket money at the beginning of the school term. Juniors were allowed to draw out two shillings and sixpence a week, which increased to five shillings for the seniors—don't forget, the British currency was made up of pounds, shillings and pence in those days!

A variety of subjects at O-level and A-level were taught at the school, we worked hard and learned much during our time there, with some of the pupils leaving school to go on to university and further education. In addition to our versatile curriculum, we were also encouraged to broaden our cultural experiences by reading or attending theatre plays. During my time in school, trips were arranged to see *The Merchant of Venice* at Stratford-upon-Avon, Gilbert and Sullivan musicals such as *The Mikado, The Pirates of Penzance* and *Trial by Jury.*

We went to see a pantomime *Cinderella* and The Crazy Gang at Oxford. The Crazy Gang comprised of a group of British entertainers and included: Bud Flanagan, Chesney Allen, Jimmy Nerve, Teddy Knox, Charlie Naughton, Jimmy Gold, and Eddie Gray. The show was hilarious and we all really enjoyed it. On one occasion we were invited to listen to the *Messiah* at the Parish Church of St Nicolas in Newbury. Our seats were near the orchestra, which was very considerate of the organisers to do, as it helped us enjoy the evening so much more. It was truly an exhilarating experience.

As much as I enjoyed these outings, I was much keener on sporting activities and enjoyed playing hockey, table-tennis, rounders, tennis, badminton, netball, and cricket. I used every opportunity to partake in these activities, whenever I found time. I remember an occasion during my holiday at Butlins in North Wales, when I wandered into a hall where people were playing table tennis. As I was watching their games, one of the players came over and asked me if I wanted to play a game. Not needing to be asked twice, I accepted with delight. I told her my name but did not catch what her name was because of the background noise. However, I really enjoyed playing with her and she invited me to come to the hall the next morning for another game—I went every day!

After we parted, I sat down to watch the other players and, after a while, a spectator sitting next to me asked which player was Diane Rowe. I looked at him and told him that I did not know. I knew who Diane Rowe was, of course but was surprised to find out that she was in my holiday resort. What would she be doing there? Later, as I got up to leave, the lady that I had been playing against called out saying 'See you tomorrow, Jean.' The spectator who was sitting next to me turned towards me and said 'I thought that you did not know which one was Diane Rowe!' I felt so silly for not catching my opponent's name when we were introduced. Still, I was elated that I had been playing table tennis with Diane Rowe, who, along with her twin sister, Rosalind was the World Ladies Double Champions in 1951.

As befitting my sporty and rather daring attitude, I was keen to learn to drive. So, I joined the Car Club in my last year at the school and learned how to drive an old Ford. We had driving lessons in the school grounds mostly in front of the manor. As the old Ford was not suitable for driving on public roads, the next move was to learn how to drive the school

Land Rover. Now, this vehicle was quite different to drive compared with the old Ford, as most of you will know, but we all made good progress and soon it was time to move on to the public roads—I really enjoyed the experience. It was fun for the most part, even though the lessons were taken very seriously. We had to look after the old Ford and, believe me I was out of my depth where the maintenance was concerned—I was happy to leave that aspect of driving instruction to my fellow club members, who seemed to know a lot about cars.

FOUR

A Sudden Loss, Too Young

Although my memories of Mary Hare Grammar School were mostly happy, one experience overshadowed my stay there— I lost my mother on 5th May 1954 when I was just thirteen years old and in form II. Mrs Askew the headmaster's wife and my form teacher at the time, broke the news to me in the headmaster's study and explained that my mother had died following a short illness. I was shocked, for I did not even know that she was ill. It was decided that, along with a school friend, we would spend the afternoon in Newbury, under the supervision of the school matron. The matron asked me if there was anything special that I would like to do—we went for a walk alongside the River Kennet, just as my mother and I did when she came to see me at half-term. I retraced our path; I struggled to accept that my mother was truly gone. I could not believe that I would never see her again. I kept hoping that someone would come along and say that it was a mistake but I knew that was not going to happen. We returned to the school in time for tea and, by then, everyone in the school knew that I had lost my mother.

During the evening, a senior girl called Barbara came over to talk to me and keep me company while everyone was doing their homework. It was a great comfort that she told me that my father would be coming to see me the following Saturday. I cried a lot during the night, although I did not disturb the other girls. The girls' matron was really kind and came in several times during the night to check on me. I was told that I did not have to attend lessons for the rest of the week, but I felt that I would cope better if I went back to school and socialized with my friends, all of whom were very supportive.

When my father arrived the following Saturday morning, I told him that I wanted to go home for a few days so that I could go to my mother's funeral. For some reason, he did not agree and I remember him saying that I would be better off staying at school. Apparently, the headmaster did not agree that I should go home either. I was adamant that they should allow me to go home for a few days so that I could go to the funeral and finally the headmaster agreed, as I promised to return to school the following Thursday.

After packing a small bag, my father and I travelled back home to Scarcliffe. There were so many questions that I wanted to ask my father but the timing was never right. The funeral was the following Tuesday at St Leonard's Church. I wanted to go so much, but my father, unbeknownst to me, had arranged for a friend of the family to take a group of children, including me, to Pleasley Vale instead. I was devastated because my father told me the morning of the funeral that I would not be attending. Looking back, I could have insisted on attending my mother's funeral, but my father had a very quick temper and I really could not deal with his anger at this particular time. Perhaps, I was a little afraid of him though I am not sure if he ever understood why I wanted to come home for a few days. By denying me the funeral attendance, I felt that he had robbed me of a chance to say goodbye to my mother and it affected me for many years. I visited my mother's grave the next morning with Auntie Ruth before returning to school the next day as promised. It was great to be back at school with my friends.

The weekend following the funeral, the heats for Sports Day were held. As I wanted to do well, instead of confronting my loss, I put all that on one side as I concentrated on qualifying for the finals. Sports Day eventually arrived and you could feel the buzz and excitement in the air, as the pupils in their appropriate House uniforms marched down to the Sports Field. The events took place one after another, as the pupils and spectators cheered their respective teams on. After all the events were completed and the winners were presented with their medals or prizes, the Champions with the Hindle Challenge Trophy led their respective Houses back to the manor.

Braidwood House came second and when Mrs Askew, the headmaster's wife, came up to my father, remarking on how proud he must be with my achievements on the sports field—I was taken aback when he simply stated that I could have done a lot better. I know that my mother would have been very proud of me. It was half-term and I realised that, when my father departed for home, there were not going to be anymore day trips to places such as Windsor Castle and sightseeing in London as was a custom for me and my mother. As sad as I was at this realisation, I was happy to stay at school at half-term because we had lots of fun and day trips were arranged for us.

When I returned home for the summer holidays, I soon realised that my relationship with the rest of the family had changed. We were practically like strangers and did not know what to say to each other. The reason for our awkwardness with each other was probably that I had changed and was more comfortable being with deaf people rather than hearing people. Hearing aids and lip-reading do make conversations easier but when talking to members of the family, I often had to rely on lip-reading to fill in the gaps. However, it is easy to make mistakes because some words are difficult to recognise. What people do not recognise is that there is a lot of guesswork involved in lip-reading, and it can be very tiring. It became apparent that, as I walked into the house and said 'Hello' to them, they would acknowledge me and then start talking between themselves again. This attitude made me feel embarrassed and uncomfortable and I would wonder when I could leave without appearing rude. It was not the same as when my mother was alive.

Returning home to an empty house was so different without my mother being there. My father was a fitter at Shirebrook Colliery and he wanted me to go to relatives while he was at work. I refused at first because I wanted to stay at home and go for walks with Laddie, visit Auntie Ruth and Uncle Harold or Uncle Ken and Auntie Mary. Uncle Ken was a headmaster at a school in Sheffield and his wife, a teacher at a local senior school in Bolsover; they would often take me out visiting places such as Dovedale, Haddon Hall, Chatsworth House, Bolsover Castle, Bakewell, and Matlock. The relationship with my father had changed and he was no longer the father figure that he once was. I attended two deaf schools, the first one being the Maud Maxfield School at Sheffield and then the Mary Hare Grammar School, a boarding school in Newbury, Berkshire.

Still, attending two deaf schools gave me a sense of belonging to a deaf community which gave me a 'deaf identity'—being partially deaf was second nature to me. My cousin, Pat told me that I had a speech impediment, but she was able to understand what I was saying and that my speech improved a lot while I was at the two deaf schools.

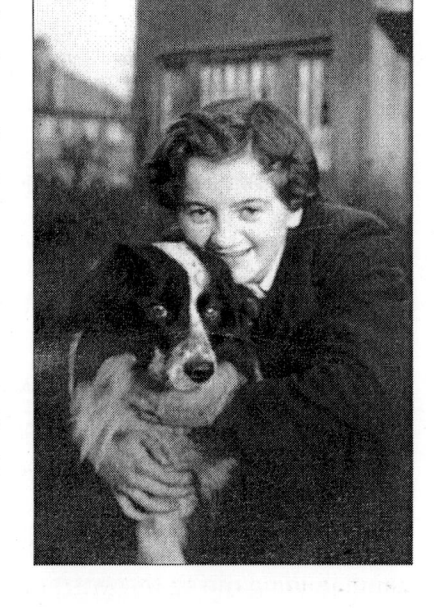

When I was at home, I would spend much of my time with Auntie Ruth and Uncle Harold, who lived in the village, as well as with Uncle Ken, my mother's brother, who taught me a lot about photography. Still, I would spend most of my time with my dog, a faithful companion called Laddie. I loved going for walks around the woods with Laddie and seeing the wild flowers. I particularly liked the wood anemones, bluebells, and daffodils although the woods were filled with many more varieties. Bluebells massed together look purple under the trees, but close up are a true clear blue. The violets that like shady places, especially under bushes and trees, are lovely, too. My Auntie Ruth often came with me and showed me many places around Scarcliffe where wild flowers could be found. I also enjoyed spending time at the brook, where I would dip my feet in the cold water while Laddie dashed around following scents. It was so peaceful and tranquil, I loved it.

Jean and Laddie.

It was while I was at the Mary Hare Grammar School, aged about fourteen, that I discovered that I could not see in the dark as well as my friends could. I had been over at the gym one night, playing badminton. At the end of the session, I went to change, suddenly realising that I was the last one to leave. As I walked out of the changing rooms, I found that all the outside lights had been switched off. I needed to get across the courtyard to the entrance to the school but could not see where I had to go—I decided to feel my way round, as it was not possible for me to walk straight across the courtyard as I could not see where I was going—everything was so black.

Fortunately, one of my friends saw me and got hold of my hand, guiding me to the entrance. He asked me what the matter was and I explained that I could not see where I was going because it was so dark. The puzzled expression on his face told me that I had a problem with my eyesight. I realise now that I could have been suffering from night-blindness for several years before finding out practically by chance. I felt a bit silly about saying that I could not see in the dark, as I was not sure that anyone would believe me. So, I told the girls' matron that I thought that there was something wrong with my eyes. An eye test was arranged for me and though the optician found no abnormalities in my eyes, he did prescribe some glasses for me, saying that I did not need them but they may keep me happy! My father was furious with me because he believed that he had paid out for something that I did not need. To be fair, he had every right to be annoyed, as the glasses did not address my problem and thus, I did not need them. It seemed as if the school was not aware of Usher syndrome at that particular time, or it could have been my fault for not explaining in more detail that I could not see in the dark. Personally, I feel that it would have made no difference.

Although my problems persisted, I managed to hide them well, as I did not feel that anyone would be particularly sympathetic—I did tell my best friend, Margaret that there was something wrong with my eyes but did not know what. During this time, I even went abroad with the school. We travelled to the Rhineland in Germany and Paris in France. I can remember seeing the Mona Lisa at the Louvre, the Eiffel Tower, and the Sacré-Coeur Basilica (Basilica of the Sacred Heart). We went out on a night trip once to see the famous landmarks, such as the Arc de Triomphe, all lit up. I did not see much as I was too busy concentrating on following some of my school friends as I was so worried about losing contact with them due to my limited night vision. No one could have been happier than I was when we arrived back at the hotel—it was a horrific experience and I was so pleased when it was all over. It was the same when the school had their annual fire practice in the middle of the night during the summer term. As, during this exercise, all lights would be switched off, I had to follow the other girls out of the dormitories, down the back stairs, across the courtyard and enter the old gym where the headmaster would be waiting to do a head count. I would follow the reverse procedure on the way back to our dormitories but this time the lights would be on although there were still some dark areas.

If only my mother was still alive, she would have listened and believed me and taken me to see a doctor and then persisted

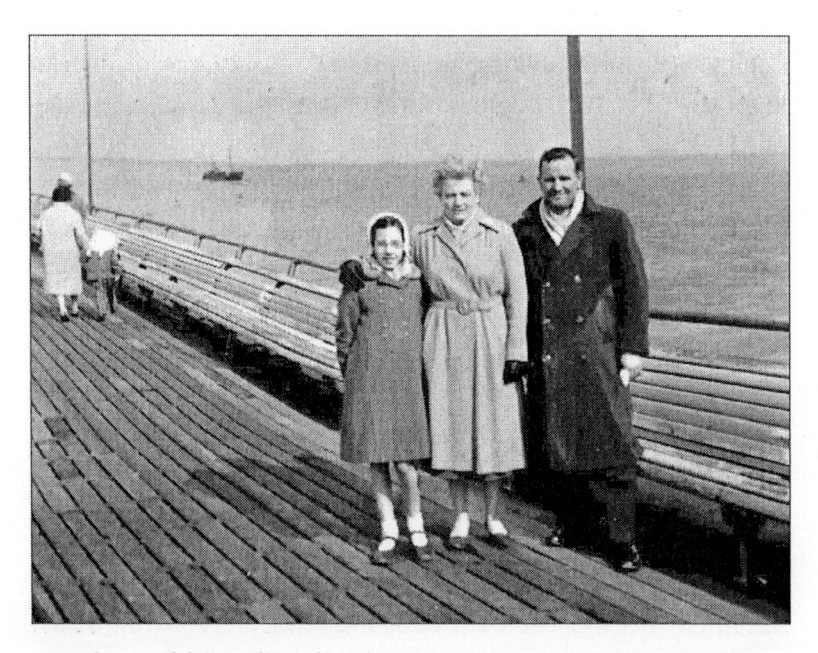

Rosalyn, Hilda and Dad.

in finding the right kind of help for me—she was a wonderful lady. However, she had died the year before and I felt truly alone. I mentioned the problem to two other people but they did not want to know, probably thought that I was seeking attention! During the school holidays, I decided to make an appointment to see the family doctor, who arranged for me to have an eye test to see if there were any abnormalities in my eyes. Returning to the surgery about two weeks later, I was told that I had to see another doctor, as the doctor that I saw previously was ill. On entering the room, I saw the doctor was seated at his desk and, while he continued to write, he told me not to be silly as no one could see in the dark. As he did not say anything else I walked out of the room, glancing at him before closing the door—he was still at his desk writing. I had no idea what to do next, as I knew that I could not see in the dark as well as I should, and recognised that there was a problem with my eyesight. Still, not a single person was willing to take me seriously.

As if that was not enough, I was in for another shock. In 1956, about a week before I was due to go on a school holiday to the Rhineland in Germany, I received a letter from my father, informing me that he was getting married to Hilda who, with her daughter Rosalyn, had visited the school a few weeks earlier. The marriage was to take place on Saturday, 14th July while I was on holiday in Germany. When they visited the school, Hilda was introduced to me as a friend of Auntie Polly and Uncle Jack, who were visiting the school as well. What my father did not seem to know was that I already knew of his relationship with Hilda, as, when I was showing them around the school, we saw the boys' matron who asked if the little girl was my sister. As I started to explain who Rosalyn was, in the background, I heard my father murmur, 'No, but it will not be long.' It was obvious to the boys' matron that I did not know, and this was probably the reason why she reported the conversation to Mrs Askew, the headmaster's wife, who discussed it with me and asked me to let her know when I heard anything more from my father. How did I feel? To be honest, my father could not have done a more efficient job in letting me know that he did not want me at the wedding.

Looking back at the course of events, I believe that my father met Hilda the previous February, having courted her before he met my mother. I have been unable to understand why he failed to tell me that he had met someone, as he had many opportunities to do so, instead of leaving it to about one week before the wedding to let me know.

I returned home after the holiday in Germany, wondering what was in store for me. I was rather surprised to find that my father and Hilda were still on their honeymoon and that I was to stay with an aunt, who lived in Glapwell—I wanted to stay with Auntie Ruth and Uncle Harold. I created a bit of a stir, albeit not on purpose. When I got off the train at Chesterfield, I noticed that Uncle Ken, who should have been meeting me, was not there. I waited, but as he still did not turn up, I decided to make my own way to Scarcliffe. On arriving at Scarcliffe, I went to see Auntie Ruth and Uncle Harold, who were delighted to see me. It was then that I was told that I should have gone to the family home down East Street, where my aunt was waiting for me. I agreed to do as I was told, asking to have something to eat first, as I was starving. I told Uncle Harold and Auntie Ruth about the holiday and how much I had enjoyed it. When Auntie Ruth and I finally arrived at the family home in East Street, we were surprised to find everyone in a panic. Apparently, Uncle Ken was waiting for me in Sheffield, instead of Chesterfield, and had reported me missing to the Railway Police. Still, as they say, all's well that ends well!

I returned home on the day that my father and Hilda were due back—shocked to find nothing that belonged to my mother in the house. Her photographs, jewellery and her lovely needlework had just disappeared as if she had been erased from my life. It was a difficult time for me as I felt that I had been stripped of everything regarding my lovely mother and that

I had nothing left. I would not have expected Hilda to have my mother's furniture, but I would certainly have expected some, if not all, of my mother's personal things to be in my bedroom for me to decide what I wanted to keep. In private, I confronted my father and asked him where my mother's personal things were. He asked me what I wanted and I gave him a list. I should have really asked for everything as, a few days later, he gave me everything that I asked for. I insisted on being told who cleared out the house, as amongst my mother's personal items that were kept in a cupboard after she had died, I had found some letters addressed to my father and me that he received when my mother died. I wanted to know where they were and why he had not shown them to me. He did not know that I had found them hidden in the cupboard and had read them all, the fact is that my father kept them from me and probably destroyed them. It saddens me that my two daughters, Anthea and Sharon, never had the chance to read those letters—and to find out what other people thought of my mother, their grandma. There were some lovely letters and my daughters would have enjoyed reading them.

Here I was with a new stepsister, ten years younger than I was, and a new stepmother, whom I barely knew. It must have been difficult for them too. I respect Hilda for telling me that she did not expect me to call her mother, suggesting that I simply call her Hilda instead. I appreciated that, but it did not stop me feeling like a stranger in my own home, even though it had not really been home for me since my mother passed away. I was unhappy for a long time, as I felt that my father was pushing me to one side now that he had a new wife and a young stepdaughter. I became very unsettled and there were times when I felt that I was a lodger in the house. It was not long after this that my father told me that I was the biggest disappointment of his life. As he never told me why he felt this way, I wondered if the reason was because I was a girl and not a boy, or because I was deaf. What I do know was that it was never the same between us after he said those cruel words.

FIVE

The Hearing World

Soon, it was time to contemplate the future, which entailed leaving the Deaf World and entering the Hearing World. I do apologise for using the terms 'Deaf World' and 'Hearing World,' but it is the only appropriate way of describing my circumstances at that time. At this point, I had attended two schools for the deaf, one being a boarding school, thus all my friends were deaf, as I had no hearing friends left at home as they had all gone their separate ways and made some new friends. After much consideration, I decided to return home due to my eyesight problems. I found employment as a laboratory assistant at Robinson and Sons Ltd, a local firm that specialised in surgical dressings and boxes. I also enrolled as a day release student at the local Technical College where I found it very hard to cope. I could not hear or understand what the lecturers were saying and often did not know what I had to do.

I eventually realised that, like it or not, deafness was a disability, albeit an invisible one, though some deaf people do not regard deafness as a disability—just a way of life. I felt cut off, unhappy and isolated. Thankfully, a few of the female students began talking to me, but it was so easy to lose the thread of what they were talking about—I was certainly the odd one out. I noticed that some students would look or walk away when they realised that I was wearing a hearing aid.

There was one lecturer who did go out of his way to help me by giving me notes at the end of the lectures, explaining what he would be talking about in the next chemistry lesson, and a list of books that I should get from the library. I appreciated his help and concern. Although I faced many daily challenges and had to spend many hours making notes in order to keep up with the other students there, I did complete the course, successfully.

I was very happy living in the Deaf World, but on entering the Hearing World, it was not long before I realised that I was not as well prepared as I would have liked to have been. I had to accept that I had many daily challenges to face that many hearing people do not experience. Still, I was determined and fully convinced that it was up to me to make a success of the final transition into the Hearing World. I can say in all honesty that my attendance at the two schools for the deaf was the only time that I felt that I really belonged to a 'group'. There were many times when I felt left out of group conversations with hearing people and was left feeling isolated. I admit that I prefer one to one conversations, as they allow me to understand most of what is being said. Still, I appreciate that some hearing people feel uncomfortable when a deaf person is lip-reading them.

Having night-vision problems made walking in poorly-lit areas extremely difficult. To try to address this issue, I would look for a guiding line, such as a wall, kerbs, some street lights, or even follow someone and hope that we do not collide. They were not good ideas, really, because it was certain that I would bump into something or someone or even trip over a kerb, but it was the only thing that I could do at that time when out on my own at night. The bus station was some distance away from the Technical College and, if I did not catch the 9.00p.m. bus, I would miss the connection at Bolsover, having to wait another hour for the next bus. To avoid the long wait in the darkness, I started walking out of the lectures a bit earlier to ensure that I caught the 9.00p.m. bus to Bolsover. By doing this, I was also able to miss the crowd of students rushing out of the buildings, which also made it unsafe for me.

I joined Robinson's Sports and Social Club and one of my work colleagues asked me to join in with her group of friends. They turned out to be a great crowd and made me very welcome. We went dancing, played hockey, table-tennis and I joined the Music Club that was run by my friend, Rosy. I did not hide the fact that I was hearing impaired or that I suffered from night-vision problems. My openness meant that I was well looked after when out at night. Still, I eventually stopped going dancing because I found it difficult to cope with the low and flashing lights. I also avoided social gatherings that went on until late at night, unless I was told that transport would be available for me. However, as many of my friends were car owners, I was not short of offers and did not have to miss out of fun.

People with Usher syndrome face enormous challenges in life and that just happens to be the cause of my problems— unknown to me at this particular time. Trying to fit in with a hearing society in a world that revolves around being able to hear and see is very challenging and the journey can be

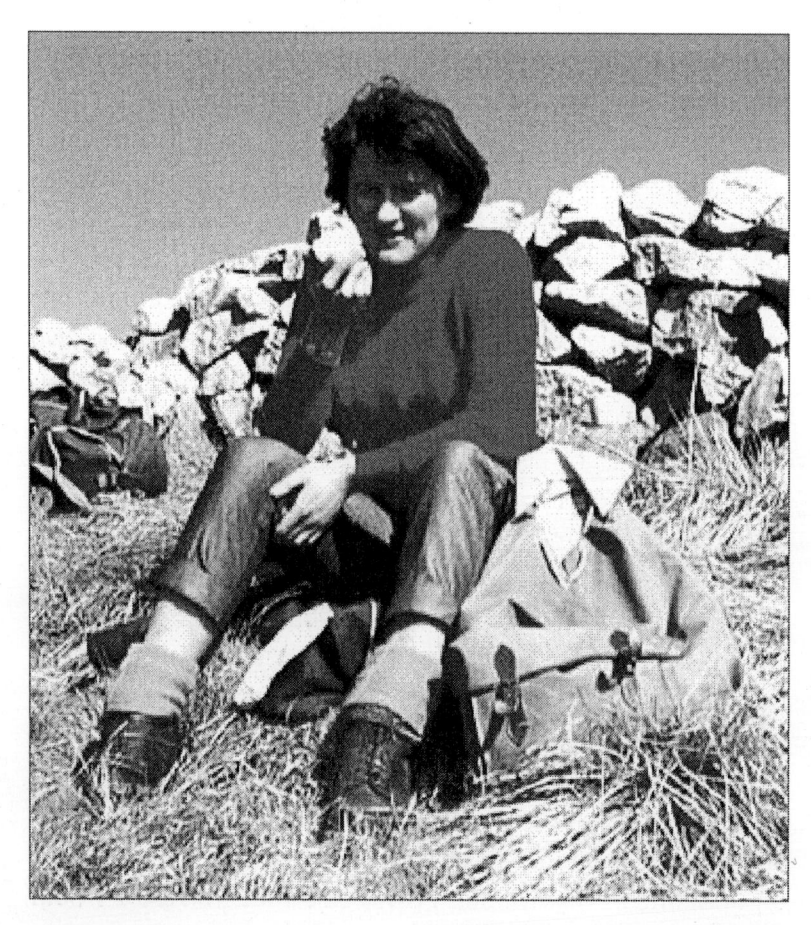

Jean hiking

a very tough one. At this time, I was only aware of my partial deafness and the fact that I have difficulties seeing in the dark—I did not know then, that I was gradually losing my sight due to a rare disease called Retinitis pigmentosa (RP). Rosy, my hearing friend was, and still is, my best friend and I will always be grateful to her for making it easier for me to interact with hearing people. It was the best thing that I ever did, joining Robinson's Sports and Social Club as it enabled me to meet other people who had similar interests and who were hearing. I made many new hearing friends.

On free days, which usually meant Sundays only, I went hiking with friends in the lovely Derbyshire Peak District. Sometimes, there would be just four of us, or as many as ten. We went camping as well and I particularly enjoyed our holiday in Pendeen near St Ives in Cornwall. There were four of us—Enid, Yvonne, Mavis, and me. People in the village made us very welcome and one very kind lady who lived at the end of the lane made us an enormous Cornish pasty, which was delicious.

When we went to the local on the first night of our holiday, we sat outside, talking to an elderly man, who really enjoyed telling us stories about the old days. The elderly man was very entertaining. Although it is likely that he started making the stories up as he went along, he was very happy to keep us company and we enjoyed talking to him.

The next night, we called at the pub again, had a chat with our elderly friend and ordered our glasses of local cider. We stayed outside, as it was a lovely evening and there seemed to be a large crowd inside. That night, two groups of young men were singing songs and attracting a lot of attention. One group was local and the other from Wales, and we know that the Welsh have a good reputation for singing. Apparently, we were noticed by the Welsh singers, as during the evening, the bartender came out with a round of drinks for us, noting that it was supplied by their rival group. The other group,

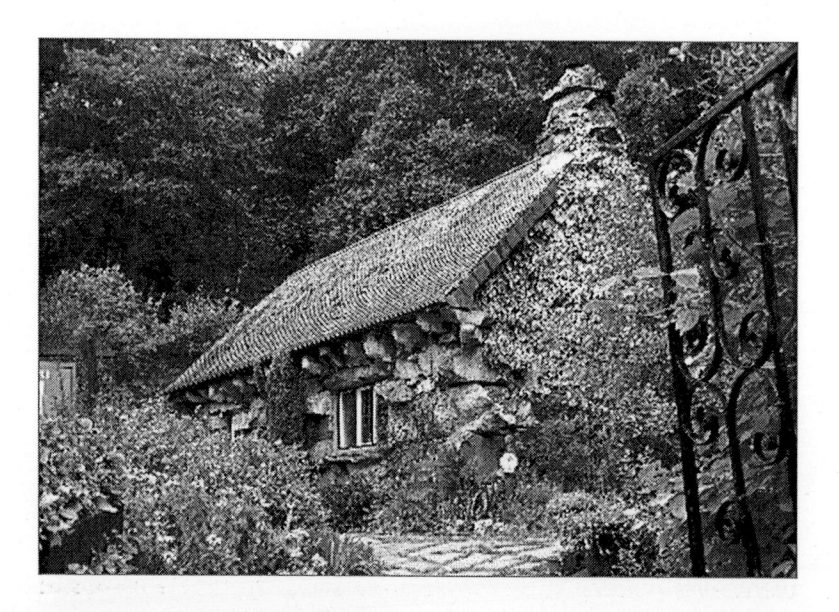

The Ugly House in North Wales

not wanting to be outdone, did the same. Three glasses of local cider each was a bit too much, but I was not completely blotto and we did find our tent, even though it was about a mile away! The next day, we went to Penzance and sailed off to the Isle of Scilly, hoping that some fresh air would clear our heads and do us good!

We went to the local every night and had a fabulous time, but we always called upon the elderly gentleman, who looked forward to seeing us and telling us some more tales of the old days. On our last night there, we were invited to the village dance. When we explained that we had no suitable attire to wear, they would not take no for an answer. At their request, we took our hiking boots off and danced in our thick yellow socks. Needless to say, we were not short of dancing partners! At the end of the evening, as we could not find our boots, we were told to sit in the middle of the dance floor and that our boots would be found for us. True to form, four pairs of red boots, and all size six, and all tied together with numerous knots, were shortly produced to us. The crowd of people there cheered and clapped while we tried to sort them out—it was a wonderful holiday and we had a fabulous time.

Another year, Mavis and I went camping in North Wales. We went on our scooters and travelled all over North Wales. The scenery was wonderful and it was a fascinating holiday. Castles, churches, gardens, Bangor, Anglesey, Bala Lakes—we went everywhere and saw all of it! We stayed at a campsite at Betws-y-coed, which is surrounded by two rivers, trees and mountains. From there, we ventured out for long walks visiting the Fairy Glen, Miners Bridge, Swallow Falls and so much more. We saw 'The Ugly House' and I found it to be full of character—I loved it! The garden was, although a bit wild, truly wonderful and it fitted in with the house. In my view, it was not ugly at all.

I liked my scooter but it did have the tendency to break down at the bottom of hills, which left me with the problem of pushing it all the way to the nearest garage. As luck would have it, I nearly always had to push it back up the hill. Eventually, I got fed up with it and decided to save up for a car—my dream was to own a sports car.

SIX

At last, a diagnosis!

Being unable to see in the dark was increasingly causing me problems and I knew that I should go and see a specialist, but I kept putting it off because of what happened the last time I saw my General Practitioner. Eventually, I decided to make an appointment to see a different GP at the same surgery. It was a struggle to see things at night even in rooms with low lighting. For example, one problem I had was when travelling home at night. Although the bus-stop was outside the family home I had problems getting to the back of the house in the dark. I worked out that if I made sure that I got off the double-decker bus before anyone else did, I would have time to dash to the gate which was only a few metres away and down the path to the back of the house before the double-decker bus set off again.

The nearest street light was about forty-six metres away so it was really dark, but the lights from the double-decker bus did help a lot. Unfortunately, it did not always work out, as there were times when I ended up on the front garden or the neighbour's garden instead and became disorientated and did not have a clue of my whereabouts. How I wished that we had a small garden at the front of the house instead of a large one. Still, I have been lost in other places as well, even when I was using the powerful torch that Uncle Ken gave me—it can be very scary and frightening especially when you do not know where you are and everything is so black. Another incident was when I fell down some steps when entering a restaurant, I do not know why I missed the steps but it was a painful experience. I desperately wanted to know what was wrong with my eyes—I wanted a diagnosis and I felt that I could not go on like this any longer without knowing what was wrong with my eyes.

It was not until I was twenty-five that Retinitis pigmentosa (RP) was finally diagnosed. Even then, the process did not go smoothly and required my going to see the General Practitioner and explaining that I would not leave the premises until he promised to make an appointment for me at the hospital regarding my eyes. After examining my eyes and asking questions about my eyesight, the GP closed the blinds and started asking me if I could see the door handle, wash basin, clock and other things scattered around the room. I am not proud to say that all my answers to his questions were 'no' when they should have been 'yes', considering that closing the blinds did not make the room dark and I could see relatively well in daylight.

Still, I was desperate to get an appointment to see a specialist at a hospital and I think the GP realised this. The GP agreed to make an appointment for me, but made it clear that it was purely to appease me. I did not care whether he believed me or not, as I was so happy to be finally going to see a consultant at the local hospital. At the hospital, atropine drops were administered into my eyes to make the irises open wider, so that the consultant could have a good look at the back of my eyes. After the examination, the consultant told me to make an appointment to see my own GP in two weeks' time. On my next visit to the

GP regarding the report from the hospital, the first thing that he did was to apologise, after which he told me that I had Retinitis pigmentosa, a condition for which there was no cure and that it would eventually lead to blindness. I could not believe that I was going blind. This was the last thing that I expected to hear, so I asked for a second opinion. I asked for a private consultation so that I could ask questions, still, it only served to confirm that I had Retinitis pigmentosa.

Yes, I cried a lot, but that was surely a natural thing to do in such circumstances. Crying is nothing to be ashamed of, at least it helped me to get rid of some pent up emotions. I mourned for a while, knowing that this condition would change my life. Indeed, the first thing that I did was to give up driving. I was always planning to buy my father's car, an Austin A40. Now, I knew that this was not going to happen. It was the correct decision, for I certainly did not want to be responsible for any fatal accidents, and I was aware that I would not be able to drive the car at night. Nowadays, I believe that, in order to obtain a driving licence, people with Retinitis pigmentosa or any other eye condition, should undergo more stringent tests before being allowed to drive on the public roads.

About six months later, I was at an all-time low. I was feeling exhausted, isolated and unwanted. I did not want well-meaning family members to overprotect me—that was the last thing I wanted. Still, I desperately needed someone to sit and talk to me about the eye disease. What do you do when you have been told that you are gradually losing your sight? Where could I go for guidance? I felt alone, as I did not know of anyone who suffered from the same condition, who could at least tell me how to prepare for the future. Some friends disappeared, most probably due to feeling inadequate and embarrassed because they did not know what to say to me. I desperately needed some emotional support, but I was not getting any, not even from my father and stepmother.

I felt so ill and my head was just a mess. I was certain that it was fear and uncertainty regarding the future. With not having any support or someone to talk to, the problems intensified and it became too difficult for me to deal with the feelings as regards to a diagnosis of impending blindness especially when I had hearing loss as well. It gave me an overwhelming feeling of hopelessness. I really needed my mother but she was not there for me. I realised that my vision problems had come to a point where my everyday life became rather restricted and realised I had to make some decisions, in particular regarding the course of action I needed to take. For a while, I tried to ignore the position that I was in, but it was impossible because of constant reminders that the disease was still there. Finally, I realised that it would be better for me to know what the future held for me rather than trying to ignore it. One thing was certain—I would eventually have to adjust to a new way of life because of failing sight. Still, I hoped that it would not be that bad, as it was not possible to predict how much vision I would lose. I remembered the advice that the specialist in Sheffield gave me which was to accept that I do have a rare eye disease for which there is no known cure or treatment, to take care of myself and have as much fun as possible. Sounds good, doesn't it? This was certainly good advice and she gave me hope by remarking that I would always have some vision, whereas others predicted a gradual loss of vision leading to blindness. I did not know what to believe, and my situation was made more complicated because no one seemed to know much about this eye disease. It became important that I find the courage to accept my condition and come to grips with the situation knowing that it would bring new pressures and problems. Still, I really had to be positive, to have a strong attitude and to have faith in myself, because if I did not accept that I had a rare eye disease then I would be in the denial mode.

It was not the end of the world, for I was sure that I could still keep going; though maybe not live as I had done previously. I was finally aware that I had to sort out any of my problems on my own. For a long time, I put on a brave face, trying to pretend that I had not a care in the world, even though, deep down, I was hurting. Nowadays, I do not have the same feelings of despair as I had then. It has not been a smooth journey, but I have come to terms with my condition and have adapted to my circumstances as well as I can. I found that I could only take one day at a time. Now, I try not to worry or think of my condition, and I try to sort out the problems as they appear.

I certainly do not blame my mother and father for the situation that I am in—it is not their fault. Although I have suffered my fair share of problems, I accept that it is just one of those things that could have happened to anyone. Back then, little was known about DNA and inherited diseases, and my parents could not have known that they were carriers of genes that caused my condition. I do my best to adapt to my circumstances, such as finding new ways to do familiar things.

Back when I was diagnosed, I decided to carry on playing hockey for as long as I could. At the time, I was playing for Staveley Ladies in the Sheffield and District League, and Chesterfield Frolics, a mixed team that played friendlies and participated in hockey tournaments. Having RP, where night-blindness is one of the main symptoms, did place limitations on my social life, though I still had my circle of close friends and I will always be grateful to my hockey friends for their unfailing support during that time. Admittedly, there have been times when I found it difficult to follow conversations around me when with a group of friends because of the noise in the background. As this made it difficult for me to get involved, I would try to start a one-to-one conversation with someone nearby, which made me feel less isolated. The hockey crowd would often meet socially for a drink or arrange a party. At Easter, we would travel to Southend on Sea to take part in a hockey tournament—there was always lots of laughter and fun and I always felt at ease in their company.

I like to take part in conversations, but I do believe that hearing people do tend to feel awkward or embarrassed when in the presence of a deaf person. This awkwardness very often leads to them talking to others, practically over the top of my head, making me feel as if I am not there. I eventually accepted this and realised that it is up to me to make the effort to overcome this barrier. This attitude had a positive outcome and often led to an easier relationship. Although we tend to talk about the problems of deaf people when they enter the hearing world, we must also realise that hearing people have their problems when meeting deaf people for the first time—it's all about confidence!

Following my diagnosis, after much thought, I decided to seek new employment, not because I had become disillusioned with my current position, but rather because I wanted a new challenge. Friends and family advised me to stay where I was, some going as far as suggesting that changing my occupation would not change anything—I would still have my problems. Still, I was determined and was successful in attaining a new position, working as a medical laboratory technician in the Biochemistry Laboratory, in the Pathology Department at the local hospital. I enjoyed this work very much and found it rewarding.

I decided to apply for a council flat in Chesterfield because at times it was unbearable being under the same roof as my father—I knew that there was a long waiting list, but I was willing to wait. After about a year, I received a letter from the council asking if I still wanted a flat as one was available. I told my Aunt Ruth and Uncle Harold that I was going to live in Chesterfield. As expected, my aunt was very upset and did not want me to go. It was such a dilemma as I really wanted to go and live in Chesterfield where most of my friends lived but did not like seeing her so upset. They had been so good to me over the years and were now in their late 70s. I knew that it would not be easy for me to visit my aunt and uncle on a regular basis because of my night-blindness and the fact that Chesterfield was about eight miles and two bus rides away, and that their home was a short distance outside the village. The eventual outcome was that I decided not to accept the flat, a decision ruled by the heart rather than the head but it proved the correct decision as my uncle died in 1969 after a battle with cancer. I visited him every day while he was in hospital and when he returned home, but it was not long before he died. Aunt Ruth let it be known to me that she would like me to move in with her, but she was afraid of what my father would say. My father and Hilda would often talk about when they move into Aunt Ruth's house down the lane, but I knew that it was not going to happen.

SEVEN

Ronald, my future husband

I met Ronald, who was to be my future husband, at a hockey tournament at Rampton in Nottinghamshire. I was playing in a match during which I was hit on the head by an opposing player's hockey stick but I did not come off—it was a rough match! As I left the pitch at the end of the game, there was Ronald, waiting on the side-lines, holding a cup of sweet tea for me. Although this was our first encounter, it took a couple of years before we started courting. He knew that I was deaf and had an eye disease that could lead to blindness, as one of our mutual friends told him. Once we started going out, I explained to Ronald in more detail what it entailed, and he was very understanding. Although he was sorry that I had these problems, he told me that it would not make any difference to him and would not affect his feelings towards me. We had similar interests and we got on so well that I knew that I wanted to spend the rest of my life with him. The way he treated me, no one would ever have known that I wore hearing aids or had an eye problem, furthermore, his family welcomed me into their midst.

We talked about our future together and asked each other if our love would be strong enough to cope with the problems that my deafness and sight impairments would bring. I wondered if, back then, he realised that, being a sighted person, he would have to be very understanding of my problems and might even have to make changes to his own lifestyle if he married me. Still, despite my reservations, Ronald was adamant that it would make no difference. We talked about having children, but we were concerned about passing the eye disease on to them—I knew that it was an inherited disease. Still, after much debate, we decided that it was a risk worth taking as there was no reason to believe that Ronald could be a carrier, or that there were any records of Retinitis pigmentosa being present in family members—past or present. Nearly forty years later, I can say that we are so glad that we took the risk, as we have two wonderful daughters, Anthea and Sharon, and five wonderful grandchildren, none of whom have been affected by my conditions.

Ronald, having lived all his life in the hearing world, had no experience of deaf people—he had to learn that one of the hardest things that many deaf people, including me, face is socialising with hearing people. Ronald wanted me to meet his family, but I was terribly nervous about it, and even managed to delay the visits. Finally, one day, he would not take no for an answer! First, I was introduced to his elder sister, Mary, her husband, Bob, and their two daughters, Janet, and Anne. I was not to know that within weeks I would be helping Anne to do her chemistry and physics homework! We got on so well and Mary told me about the rest of the family while she showed me the family album. It was not long before I met the rest of the family and they were all so friendly and sociable. I am so pleased that I met Ronald's mother who was a lovely lady and so devoted to her family. It was very sad that she died a few weeks after our meeting, just two months before our wedding.

Ronald left school when he was fourteen years old and found employment at Bryan Donkin Ltd, a firm situated on Derby Road in Chesterfield, Derbyshire. He started work on 9th August 1945, as an apprentice fitter. At the age of eighteen, he was transferred to the Governor Shop, where he was trained to be a tester and eventually became Chief Governor Tester when he was twenty-eight. Ronald was a committee member of the Sports and Social Club and eventually became Vice-Chairman. Social and sporting activities organized by the committee included football, cricket, crown green bowling, Saturday night dancing, snooker, and Christmas parties for the children. He was the proud manager of Bryan Donkin's football team that played in the Chesterfield League for two seasons. I fondly remember going to some of the football matches!

Ronald's pastime was playing for Bryan Donkin's team in the Chesterfield Crown Green Bowling League, but when the club lost the ground that was situated at Boythorpe Inn, he moved to Robinsons and later to Highfield Bowling Club, where he was Club Captain for about ten years. In 1999, Ronald finally stopped playing bowls due to ill health and was later made an Honorary Life Vice-President. I can remember going to football matches at Saltergate to watch Chesterfield Town play during the football season and Derbyshire County Cricket team at Queens Park in the summer.

Ronald loved to entertain the family and children with some party tricks, where he used coins, pretending to throw the coins into the air and then finding them behind someone's ear or whatever fun place he could think of. The children loved it! Mind you, Hannah, one of the children, tried to copy him, but instead of coins she used grapes from her Granny's fruit bowl and was throwing them all over the place. Ronald had an infectious smile, he was fun loving and loved to tell jokes. There was never a dull moment when Ronald and his older brother, George were around.

We married at my village church on 25th September 1971, in presence of many family members, friends and people from the village—the church was full. I wore a full length white grosgrain satin dress and a three tier veil, which was secured by a headband—I carried pink and yellow roses. My bridesmaid was my stepsister Rosalyn, who wore a turquoise chiffon Empire line dress and carried pink carnations. Ronald's elder brother, Eddie, was the best man. The Rev. G Dickenson conducted the service and my mother's brother, Uncle Ken, played the organ. A reception was held at the Sportsdrome Club in Bolsover and we left for a honeymoon in Shanklin on the Isle of Wight.

Ronald and I enjoyed the wedding service, and I was so grateful to the Rev. G Dickenson for holding his service book in front of me, so that, by following his finger, I knew what he was saying and what I had to say. After taking our marriage vows, Ronald and I moved towards the altar for prayers. After prayers we moved back to the front of the congregation. Ronald and I signed the register in front of the entire congregation, instead of behind closed doors, in the vestry. I was pleased about this because the church was filled with family, friends and people from the village, and it was great to share that precious moment with them. I believe this was done on purpose so that I could avoid any steps on entering the vestry

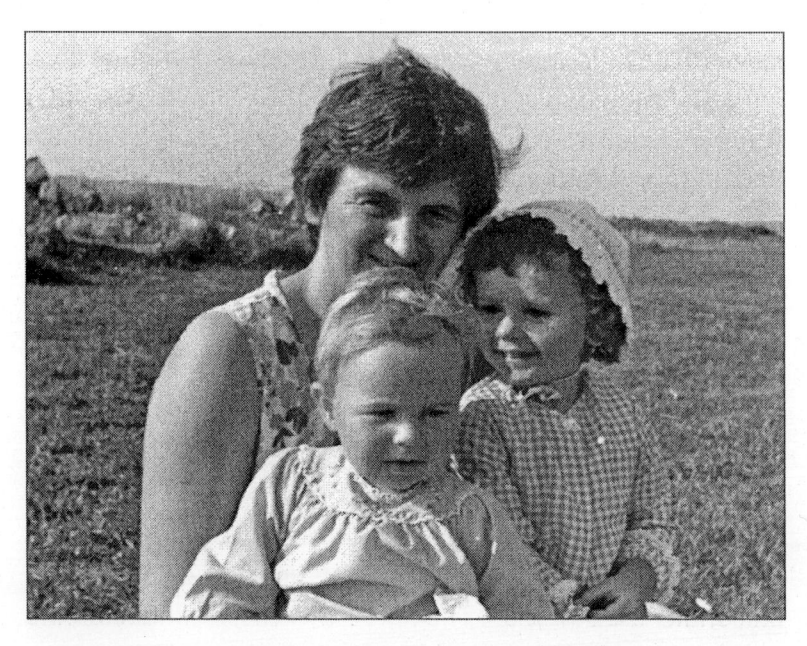

Jean with her two daughters, Anthea and Sharon.

and any other hazards that I may have had to face because of my impaired vision.

As I reflect on our beginnings, I feel compelled to tell you this delightful little story that Ronald told me when we were looking at some of my family albums. I remember, as we were looking at the photographs, Ronald recognised a lady in a photograph and asked me how I knew her. I would not tell him at first, wanting to know how he knew her, and this is what he told me. Ronald lived in St Augustine in Chesterfield and went to St Mary's School. As the school was situated on the other side of Chesterfield, he had to walk through the town. Ronald told me that when he and his friends had enough money between them, they would call at a chemist's shop on their way home from school for some hard liquorice. The lady in the shop would divide it between them so that each boy received an equal share. I told him that the lady was, in fact, my mother and he was so delighted that he had actually met my mother even though it was some years ago. Who would have thought that Ronald would one day marry this lady's daughter?

Our first daughter, Anthea was born on 25th October 1972, soon followed by Sharon, who arrived on 18th April 1974. Ronald and I decided that I should be a full-time mother instead of returning to work, as we both firmly believed that having a mother at home with the children during their formative years was very important. I was there to witness their first smile, their first tooth, and their first word—which was 'dada'—as well as their first step. These were such precious moments that I will always treasure. When they were ill, I was there to care for them, and to play, and read stories to them, but their father was the one who took them to bed and read the bedtime stories. I was there when they arrived home from school. I certainly enjoyed being a mother to Anthea and Sharon. Their father enjoyed playing games with them and singing nursery rhymes. When the girls were older and had their guitars, their father went out and bought a second-hand violin so that he could join in with them, but it was a complete disaster! Can you imagine what it was like? With the two girls playing their guitars, their father playing a violin that he did not know how to play, joined by our two family dogs howling loudly! Well that was what it was like, and it was not long before I put a stop to all that noise.

My sight problems took a back seat, as they did not seem to be affecting my everyday life. In addition, the family adapted to my circumstances over time, and were all positive about my condition. Our two girls were brought up knowing that I had a sight problem, that I had poor night vision, and that I could not hear too well unless I had my hearing aids on. They soon learned that they had to touch me on my arm if they wanted my attention. I do admit that I used to enjoy time out, as, when I took my hearing aids off, it was so peaceful and calming. When the girls wanted to talk to me, they would fetch my hearing aids and give them to me.

We lived a rather ordinary, happy life as a family. Often, we would enjoy days out to places, such as Matlock, Dovedale, Chatsworth, and Bakewell, sometimes accompanied by Uncle Ken, my mother's brother, who adored the two girls. We started going farther afield by organising excursions for family and friends and we visited Chester Zoo, Blackpool Illuminations, York, Windsor Safari Park, and London. For a number of years, we went on holiday with Ronald's sister, Pat, her husband, Francis, and their two children, Richard and Rachel, with whom we had lots of fun and laughter.

Still, on occasion, a problem due to my deafness and night-blindness would come up. I remember the time when we took the two girls to the pictures for the first time and, within minutes of the film starting, Sharon decided that she wanted to go to the toilet. My first reaction was to panic, as Ronald could not take her and, as I suffered from night-blindness, I would not be able to take her either, being unable to see where I was going. Ronald had the brilliant idea that Sharon should take me to the exit and that was what she agreed to do! He explained to Sharon that she was to hold her mother's hand and take her where it said 'Exit' and he showed her where that was. Did she take me to the exit? No, she did not. What she did instead was to lead me down a row that had no way out at the other end! Ronald realising what was happening, rescued us and took us back to our seats. Afterwards, he took Sharon to one of the lady members of the staff and asked her if she would take Sharon to the toilet. After this, we decided that, whenever we went to the cinema, we would ensure that we went with a group of friends or family members.

On occasion, I would bump into furniture at home. I would stumble over things on the floor, but this was usually when someone inadvertently moved something. I thought that I was simply being clumsy and was not unduly worried about it. When our two girls were very young they would leave toys and books around the home but that is what all young children do when playing with their toys. My husband kept telling me to stop rushing about and to take my time!

Nowadays, the first thing that I do is to scan any room that I enter and take note of where things are even if it is someone else's home that I visit regularly, as you never know if they have moved any furniture around! I will take particular care in noting where the doors are and whether they are closed, half closed, or open, as colliding with a partially opened door really hurts—I know because I have done it so many times, especially with cupboard doors!

When the girls started school, I felt a bit lost, mainly because I found that I had too much free time on my hands. So, I decided to join the Mother's Christmas Workshop which led to many other outlets. Far from ignoring my sight and hearing problems, I was gradually learning to live with the condition, instead of sitting at home and worrying about it. The experiences I had as a result of my deafness have, I am certain, helped me to face up to my visual problems as well. In particular, although it may seem a paradox, helping other people to understand my difficulties by talking about them has helped me to overcome many of my problems. One thing that I often say to my new friends is that, if they see me in town or wherever, they must tap me on my shoulder to get my attention, as I would not want them to think that I was ignoring them. Having tunnel vision makes it easy for friends to feel that they have been ignored if I do not acknowledge them. One lady did, as she knew that I had sight problems, but did not know that I was hearing impaired too. Hence, she thought that I had ignored her when she apparently spoke to me when she saw me in town. These things do happen! This lady did not speak to me for weeks, and I would never have known what had caused her to distance herself from me had it not been for her confiding to a mutual friend, who explained to her that I was deaf as well as sight impaired. The lady was horrified to realise what she had done, and could not wait to apologise to me—we both laughed about it.

EIGHT

The Social Worker

During one of my visits to the optician for my regular eye test, he advised me to contact the Social Services and even asked if he could phone someone to fetch me—he was so worried about me getting back home. My husband, Ronald, made the call to the Social Services as there was no point in me phoning because of my hearing impairment. Within a few days, a social worker for the blind came to my home. I was asked to register as a partially sighted person, but I refused on the grounds that I did not consider that I was at that stage yet. It could be that I was just being stubborn as the idea of being registered as a partially sighted person did not really appeal to me. The social worker continued to visit me, even if it was only to ask how I was, which was really kind of her. Still, as a result of our meeting, I went to help with the Talking Newspaper, where I enjoyed helping out and meeting the other volunteers.

One day while out shopping in town, I fell and badly grazed both my knees. I was pleasantly surprised when the social worker turned up at my home the next morning before going to work to see how I was doing! I had to admit that I'd had a fall although I wondered if she already knew. After a brief chat, she asked me if I would reconsider my choice of not accepting the registration—she really seemed keen to help me. I agreed to go, probably because I was feeling very vulnerable at that time. This decision, however, led to my being registered as a 'Blind Person', rather than as a 'Partial Blind Person' as expected. I was horrified and would not accept the label 'Blind Person', for, in my view, a blind person cannot see anything and I still had some vision thus, I could not see how I could be registered as a 'Blind Person'. It was just the words that were hurting me, and I am glad that the terms used nowadays are 'sight impaired' (Partially Blind) and 'severe sight impaired' (Blind)—it is a more acceptable description that does not make me feel that I am heading for the scrap heap.

Following the incident, the social worker wisely kept out of my way for a few weeks and I had no contact with her until the day that I received an invitation from the Derby Branch of the British Retinitis Pigmentosa Society of which I was a member, where I was invited to attend a meeting the next day. Their guest speaker was Mary Guest, a founder member of the Society with a special interest in people affected by Retinitis pigmentosa and deafness. I really wanted to attend, but was unfortunately unable to, as, at the time, we did not have a car. Later that day, I received a phone call from one of the volunteers who helped at Talking Newspapers, soon followed by a call from my social worker, who had arranged some transport to take me to Derby.

I enjoyed the Branch meeting and was afterwards even able to discuss my difficulties in accepting my registration as a blind person with Mary Guest. She was a great help to me and I have always appreciated the time she gave me that day. The next day, I went to help out at the Talking Newspaper again and saw my social worker, who asked if I was ready to talk. After replying that I was, I followed her to her office. After thanking my social worker for arranging the transport and apologising for my behaviour, we discussed the meeting with Mary Guest and my attitude to becoming severely sight impaired. The social worker offered me a white cane as well as a red and white cane. However, despite my acceptance of the 'label' given to me, I did explain that I would never use the red and white cane, but would accept the white cane when I was ready. I just needed time to get used to the fact that I had a dual sensory disability of hearing loss and sight loss because it was proving so hard to take it in.

The reason that I would not use a red and white cane was that I found that not many people were aware of its significance. Most people knew that a white cane indicated that the person carrying it was vision impaired, but very few knew that a red and white cane indicated that its holder was deaf as well as being vision impaired, thus I believed that I would be safer using a white cane at that particular time. I will admit that I have never used the red and white cane, even though I took it home with me. Many deaf/blind people carry a red and white cane to let people know that they have hearing and sight problems, but not many people seem to be aware of this.

People have stopped me to ask how I have managed with the white cane, albeit mostly individuals who are vision impaired themselves. A symbol cane is a short cane that can be folded and kept in a pocket or bag. When necessary, it can be brought out when in busy areas, or when crossing a road, to indicate to others that you have a visual impairment. The first white cane that I had was a guiding cane, a folding one—a straight cane that can be folded into four sections and held together by an elastic chord. The white cane is used by vision impaired people as a mobility tool and as a courtesy to sighted people. Courtesy is just as important, as carrying a white cane lets others know that you have a sight problem and warns them to be careful. I understand why some vision impaired people are reluctant to use the white cane because I did not want to use mine at first, mainly because I could not accept being registered as a blind person, and I did not wish to advertise that I had a sight problem.

The first time I went out carrying my white cane, it was not long before I folded it up and put it in my bag, explaining that I did not need it while I was with my husband, Ronald. Still, I would admit that it was just an excuse to get out of using it. It was some weeks before I went out with it again. I felt embarrassed and uncomfortable, as I was worried about being seen by family, friends, or neighbours. What would they say to me? I found that no one took any notice, but, some expressed admiration at my courage. Indeed, it did take courage to go out into town carrying a white cane for the first time. I was even told that I looked well with the white cane and I did appreciate the encouragement that I was given by my relatives and friends, but I knew that they were trying to help me to accept the white cane. Using the white cane as a mobility tool was much better than bumping into people, falling down steps, or tripping over kerbs, which probably resulted in passers-by thinking that I was clumsy.

You may be interested in how the white cane was developed, so here is a brief history! Even though blind people have been using their canes for centuries, the white cane was not introduced until after the First World War. In 1921, John Biggs of Bristol, who was a photographer, became blind after an accident and, because he was uncomfortable with the amount of traffic surrounding his home, he painted his walking stick white to make it more visible. Ten years later, Guilly d'Herbemont of France launched a national white cane movement for blind people.

I received tremendous support from the social worker and she seemed to understand not only my difficulties, but also those that most people with sight problems have to face. When I mentioned this to the social worker, she told me that, in order to help her to understand the difficulties that partially sighted and blind people have, she would perform tasks, such as having a bath, in the dark. I tried having a bath in the dark and I did not find it that easy but I did realise that you had to be very well organised in terms of knowing where everything was for it to work. Walking around the home at night with no lights on would certainly be good practice, but my husband was reluctant to let me try it. I still did, which reminds me to warn anyone deciding to have a go, to ensure that all the doors are closed, for it really does hurt when you walk into a door!

My social worker asked me if I was interested in going on a six-week swimming course. I joined other sight-impaired people at a local swimming pool—some social workers joined us as well, obviously to keep a watchful eye on us! An area, lengthwise, was cordoned off for our use and we went every Wednesday morning for about six weeks—the water was a bit warmer on Wednesday morning! After about three weeks, I asked if I could have a go at swimming a length—I had four people swimming alongside me, one at the front, behind me, on the left side and right side—one person walked alongside the swimming pool holding a long pole above me. I swam most of the way, but did not reach the other end because that was where the other sight impaired people had congregated! It was good fun and I enjoyed meeting the other people who had sight problems—it made me realise that I was not alone.

Another course that I went on was 'Health and Personal Care' at the Technical College—it was fun and I really enjoyed it, but a word of advice, do not let anyone who is severely sight impaired wash your hair—I did! We were told that we were going to work in pairs this particular afternoon and wash each other's hair. Some of the social workers turned up with extra towels and one stayed with me while my hair was washed. Yes, I got wet—very wet! This was followed by a six week cookery course and I made my very first Christmas cake. I learned how to make some corn dollies—only the simple ones and I found it to be a fascinating subject—this tradition goes back thousands of years. I practised making corn dollies with drinking straws at first before making them with corn.

One summer day, accompanied by another lady who also had sight problems, and two social workers, I went for a bike ride on the Tissington Trail. We travelled by car to Parsley Hay and then hired two tandems. This is a great way to cycle for two people of different abilities—in this case one with normal sight and one who is registered blind. We set off down the track, my social worker at the front doing all the hard work, with me just pedalling away at the back. It was a lovely warm sunny day and was perfect for cycling. The trail is thirteen miles long and runs from Ashbourne to Parsley Hay—we did not go all the way.

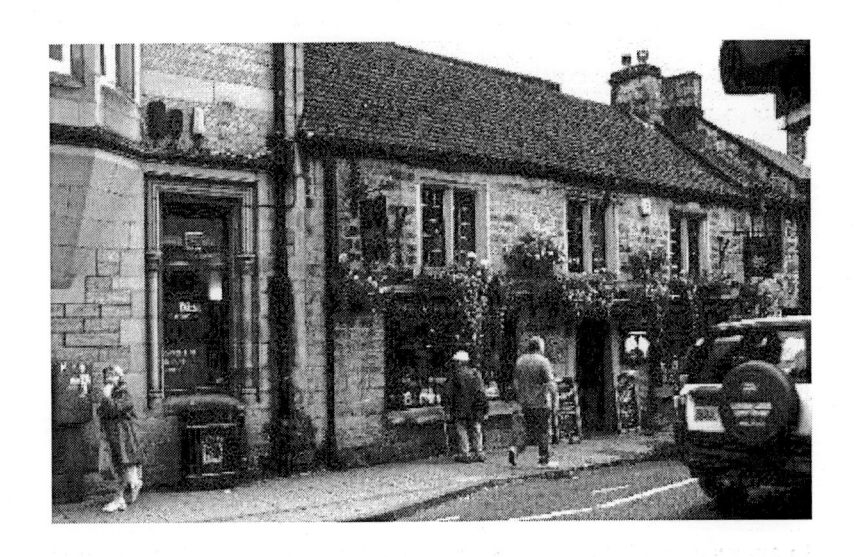

We were surrounded by beautiful countryside and it was traffic-free—it was previously an unused rail track. On our return journey, my social worker suddenly decided to stop for some reason and then turned towards me and suggested that I have a go at the front! I was not sure if I had heard her correctly! Apparently, I did, so after discussing what signals to use, we set off down the trail with me at the front! The trail was quite wide at this point, so there was no real danger of cycling off the track. Still, after a short ride, we swapped places again. After returning to the depot, we went for some lunch and then called at Bakewell to buy some Bakewell Pudding from 'The Old Original Bakewell Pudding Shop' (above). We had such a wonderful time that I took Ronald, my sister-in-law Mary, and the girls for a cycle ride the following week—we took a picnic with us too!

I have always enjoyed outdoor and sporting activities and the cycle ride was just one of many examples of fun things I did. As the girls got older and wanted more freedom to go out with their friends, it was suggested that I join Highfield Bowling Club where Ronald was already a member. I decided to apply for membership and was invited to join. I had already played bowls with Ronald when on holiday in Rhyl in North Wales and really enjoyed playing the game. The bowling club that I joined played in the Chesterfield and District Crown Green Bowling League and, though the club did not have many teams playing in the league at the time, it was not long before the club started entering more teams due to increased membership.

The club decided to have a Ladies team to play in the League— I started going down to the green most mornings to practice on my own and to get to know the green, as I really wanted to play for the team. The practice paid off as I was picked to play with Olga, who was a wonderful team player, and we played well together. As well as playing for the ladies team, I played for the club in the Saturday Singles League and the Wednesday Doubles League. I had to work hard at my game, but was able to develop a technique that worked for me. Still, I found it difficult at times, especially when playing in bright conditions and would often end up with a severe headache and feeling sick. After a few years, Ronald was ready to pack up due to health problems and I decided to leave at the same time, as I was no longer enjoying the bowling scene.

NINE

British Retinitis Pigmentosa Society

I joined the British Retinitis Pigmentosa Society in 1981. The Society was founded in 1975 by a group of people that had Retinitis pigmentosa (RP) or had a special interest in the eye disease. This group of people was disquieted by the lack of knowledge regarding Retinitis pigmentosa in the medical profession and the lack of support for people diagnosed with this condition; they were determined to do something about it so they founded the Society. Their aim was twofold: to help find a cure by raising funds for research and to provide information and support for people diagnosed with Retinitis pigmentosa and for their families. I applied for membership and, within days, received the much-awaited reply. I had waited a long time for this information, but it still did not make comfortable reading. To be honest, it was depressing, but it did answer some of my questions. When I was first told that I had Retinitis pigmentosa it was obvious then, that there was very little known about the disease, as I was basically told that I had got RP and that it leads to blindness. However, when I was diagnosed with Retinitis pigmentosa, I was not to know that this was the start of what could be a troubling journey.

Retinitis pigmentosa causes night-blindness and a gradual loss of peripheral vision because of the progressive degeneration of the retina —there is no cure or treatment available. Retinitis pigmentosa does not describe one medical condition, but a group of hereditary degenerative diseases of the retina, that lead to a gradual progressive loss of vision—the retina is a light sensitive tissue at the back of the eye. There are no outward signs on my eyes to suggest that I am severely sight impaired but a significant feature of RP is that it progresses over many years. In most cases the symptoms of RP are restricted to the eye, however, RP can be part of a disease syndrome that affects other parts of the body—the most common being Usher syndrome.

The first symptoms of Usher syndrome to appear are difficulty seeing in rooms with low light conditions, or being outdoors at dusk or in the dark, and this is commonly known as night-blindness. This is followed by a gradual loss of peripheral vision due to a slow degeneration of the rod cells that lie on the periphery of the retina. As RP progresses the field vision narrows until only the central vision remains—commonly known as tunnel vision.

When looking straight ahead, people with normal vision would be more aware of movement on both sides. For people with Usher syndrome, this vision will be considerably impaired, hence this is the reason why I bump into lamp posts, pedestrians, trip or stumble over kerbs, and steps, and why I miss seeing overhanging branches when I am out walking. This information indicated that my field vision was actually narrowing, which was why I was bumping into things, rather than as a result of my clumsiness, as I initially thought. My reading vision and colour vision were affected later. The rate at which the vision deteriorates is flexible but is generally very slow with changes occurring over years rather than months.

Tunnel vision is still not fully understood, but is assumed to be related to the malfunction in the regeneration of photoreceptor cells that are located in the retina at the back of the eye and consist of two types called rods and cones. They play an important role by providing us with our vision. The rods are responsible for the peripheral vision and the absorption of light in dim light while the cones control the central vision and colours. Basically, what I have been told is that cells die off naturally, but in people who have RP they are not replaced with new ones, as would be the case in a person with a healthy retina. A loss of rods will result in a loss of night-vision and peripheral vision, whereas a loss of cones leads to a loss of central vision and the ability to distinguish colours, resulting in a slow loss of vision.

Putting it all in a nutshell, due to the loss of side vision, meaning the area surrounding my visual field, I fail to see objects above, below and to both sides making it impossible for me to see objects unless they were directly in front of me. The combination of hearing and sight loss also made it difficult for me to realise when someone was approaching me from the side and often from the front. If you try to imagine what it is like in a supermarket when shoppers with their trolleys are approaching you in all directions you will realise how difficult it is to cope with this condition. Some people even leave their trolley unattended in the middle of the gangway and that is when I nearly always accidentally bump into a trolley. There

I am apologising, while the owner gives me a disapproving look until they see my white stick. Then it is all smiles and apologies! To avoid this issue, I push the trolley and whoever is with me holds the trolley at the front to guide it along.

There are several rare conditions where RP is associated with other problems such as deafness. They are known as Retinitis pigmentosa syndromes and are also caused by faulty genes. Usher syndrome is a genetic disorder with hearing loss and a progressive loss of vision due to Retinitis pigmentosa, and in some cases there are balance problems, too. Usher syndrome is the most common condition in the United Kingdom that affects both hearing and vision. The hearing loss is sensorineural deafness, a problem with the inner ear or the auditory nerve. Some types of Usher syndrome can affect the development of the vestibular organs in the inner ear which are responsible for balance.

People with sensorineural deafness tend to complain that people are mumbling and, though they can hear them talking, they do not understand what they are saying. It is said that the aging process is a very common cause of sensorineural hearing loss for, as we get older, the inner ear nerves and sensory cells gradually die.

Cochlear implants can help people to hear and understand speech more clearly especially if they are unable to benefit from using a hearing aid. Cochlear implants consist of: (1) A receiver which is surgically implanted in the mastoid bone behind the ear, with electrodes inserted into the cochlea which is part of the inner ear; (2) A microphone and speech processor converts sound into an electrical signal that is sent to the electrodes in the inner ear. These then stimulate the auditory nerve sending a signal to the brain, where it is perceived as sound.

There are three types of Usher syndromes—Usher syndrome type 1, Usher syndrome type 2 and Usher syndrome type 3—Usher syndrome type 1 and type 2 being the most common in the United Kingdom.

People with Usher syndrome type 1 are born profoundly deaf. Hearing aids are not usually much help for them, and sign language is used for communication. There are also severe problems with balance and sight with night-blindness usually being the first symptom to appear.

People with Usher syndrome type 2 are usually born with moderate to severe hearing loss. Balance tends to be normal. Hearing aids are found to be helpful, and many people use speech and lip-reading for communication. People with Usher syndrome type 2 may experience balance problems resulting from the combined effect of sight and hearing loss.

People with Usher syndrome type 3 are born with normal hearing and sight but problems are usually evident during their teens. By the time they are in their 40s most people with type 3 are blind and have complete hearing loss. They also develop balance problems.

There is currently no cure for Usher syndrome, but it is feasible to protect our vision and hearing and to find ways to adapt to the daily challenges of Usher syndrome.

Usher syndrome is inherited which means that it is passed from parents to their children through changed or mutated genes. The pattern of inheritance for Usher syndrome is an autosomal recessive gene and both parents must pass the faulty gene to their child for the child to have Usher syndrome. Autosomal means that both male and female can have the disorder and can pass the disorder to a child. Recessive means that a person must inherit a change in the same gene from each parent in order to have the disorder. If only one changed gene is inherited, the child will be a carrier of Usher syndrome, but will not develop the condition themselves. If a mother and father who each carry one copy of the same mutated gene—carriers of Usher syndrome—decide to have a child together, then, with each birth there is a:

✦ One in four chance of having a child with Usher syndrome.
✦ Two in four chance of having a child who is a carrier but does not have Usher syndrome.
✦ One in four chance of having a child who does not have Usher syndrome and is not a carrier

I understand that I have been hearing impaired since birth thus, I have grown up living with deafness, and the sight loss is due to RP that developed during my teens. Hence, it is not surprising that I found it difficult to come to terms with losing my sight as well. Though I have adapted to my hearing loss well and, as I have already mentioned, I have always relied on my sight to help with lip-reading. Still, it was not until much later that I realised just how much I depended upon my vision to help with communication.

A Scottish ophthalmologist, Charles Howard Usher (1865–1942) who studied medicine at St Thomas Hospital in London, received his doctorate in 1891 and remained at St Thomas Hospital, working under Edward Nettleship (1845–1913). Later, he became an eye surgeon at the Aberdeen Hospital for Sick Children, and also worked in the Aberdeen Royal Infirmary. In 1914, Charles Usher described about forty families in a survey of hearing loss and blindness. Usher demonstrated that the disease was inherited, and that parents passed the condition onto their children. His discovery was a continuation of the work done by German ophthalmologists Albrecht von Graefe and Richard Liebreich, who conducted extensive research of Retinitis pigmentosa and its link to deafness in the mid-19th century.

I have often been asked the question—which is worse, to be deaf or to be blind? I find, however, that comparing the effect of my handicaps can be rather futile. If one answers, 'It is worse to be deaf', blind people tend to become offended and vice versa. I have found over the years that the sum of my two handicaps creates a greater handicap than the problem of partial sight or partial hearing would in isolation. The combination of the two senses becomes greater because of the impact that they have on each other, often making it hard for deaf/blind people to benefit from services for the deaf or services for the blind. It must be very hard for healthy people to imagine what it is like to be blind or deaf or even deaf/blind. Still, hearing and sighted people should consider what their friends and relatives with these two handicaps might have done, if they had not been so handicapped. For instance, the friend might have been a good pilot, a doctor, a banker, or even a professional cricketer. On the other hand, they have to appreciate that the individual may well have gained tremendous practical skills or insights because of their handicaps.

Helen Keller, the well-known American deaf/blind legend, was asked which one of her two disabilities she considered to be the worse. She explained that she would rather be blind as with hearing, she would still be able to have conversations with people around her and would not feel isolated.

> 'Deafness is a much worse misfortune... Blindness cuts us off from things, but deafness cuts us off from people.'

We enjoyed fundraising for the British Retinitis Pigmentosa Society (BRPS), collecting at the local supermarkets and in Chesterfield town centre. We also arranged social activities such as 'Bring and Buy' and 'Coffee mornings.' I had a group of friends who gave me tremendous support, and I know that without their help, I would not have been able to do it. Robinson's Operatic Society did a show for us once and I invited Lynda Cantor, a founding member and secretary of the British Retinitis Pigmentosa Society, as well as Elaine Harris, who had a regular slot every Sunday on Radio Sheffield, to join us. We had a brilliant time, which continued well into the early hours at our home.

Our family went to several conferences and meetings and it was good to meet other people who experienced the same problems. We also once went to a 'Weekend Away', which was just for people diagnosed with RP and deafness and their families. Mary Guest asked me if I would give a short speech about how I coped with RP and deafness and, noting my reluctance, explained that there would be four of us talking about how we coped, with only about twenty people in the audience. After she added that the speech should only last for about ten minutes, I decided that I would do it, but soon realised that you can say a lot in ten minutes. However, apparently Mary miscalculated, as there were a lot more than twenty people there and, for once, I was glad that I had tunnel vision, as it meant that I could not see many of them! My speech lasted ten minutes, and I took a corn dolly that I had made to show them.

At the 'Weekend Away' I saw some members who had Usher syndrome being led around by escorts or possibly their family or friends. To communicate, the interpreters would sign on their hands using the Deaf/Blind Alphabet Manual. The members appeared to be very cheerful and I admired them very much and their attitude did have a lasting effect on me. I believe it was while I was there that I obtained a copy of the Deaf/Blind Alphabet Manual. It did make me realise how important it was for deaf/blind people to be able to communicate with other people especially family and friends. The Deaf/Blind Alphabet Manual is an easy to learn tactile method of feeling along with sign language and finger spelling, as these are extremely important for people with a dual sensory impairment. I am confident that technology which is advancing rapidly will continue to provide help for people with hearing and sight problems. During the 'Weekend Away' I had a go at doing some Braille and looked at some other examples such as Moon—I found it fascinating. When I returned home, I asked my social worker if I could learn how to do Braille and I did, even though I did not really need it at that time. Still, you never know, it may be useful one-day!

People who are deaf/blind face severe difficulties in their lives and because there is no cure or treatment available at this present time, those affected still face progressively losing their sight and hearing. Deaf/blindness is a dual sensory loss of both hearing and sight and Usher syndrome is one of the main causes of deaf/blindness. Most deaf/blind people have some useful residual vision or hearing, very few are totally deaf or totally blind. I am severely deaf and severely sight impaired but do not regard my condition to be severe enough to be labelled deaf/blind at this present time. Still, I do not habitually label myself and so do not identify or define myself as deaf/blind because I do not feel that way inclined. I do, however, accept that one day I may have to consider myself as deaf/blind, but not yet.

Other problems include difficulties with adjusting to different lighting conditions, such as when I enter a brightly lit room or go outside when it is very bright. For a short time I am unable to see anything until my eyes gradually adjust. It is just as bad when I enter a room after being outside in bright light. However, it is easier to manage, as I can wait until my eyes have adjusted to the new conditions before starting to move around. To help to protect my eyes, I started to wear red lenses, as they are recommended for people with my condition—due to the high contrast that they provide, as well as enhancing the background—they are ideal for bright and overcast days. I have been told that, in some cases of RP, glare from bright lights is a problem, though some people do not experience this until the advanced stages of the disease. There have been several occasions when I have been asked if there was a medical reason why I was wearing red lenses or if I was wearing them for cosmetic reasons. I can remember one very young lady looking very disappointed after I explained that it was because I had an eye disease and here I thought that I was going to start a new trend!

It disturbed me to find that I would eventually become more dependent on my hearing aids, as my sight would eventually deteriorate to the point that it would be difficult to rely on my increasingly narrow vision for lip-reading. In the early stages of the disease, the vision loss occurs very slowly and so it is possible to adjust without realising that there had been any change. There were occasions when I mentioned to my husband, Ronald, that I felt that my eyes had changed a bit, but more often than not, he had already noticed. During one of my regular visits to the optician, it was found that I had a slow growing cataract forming on both eyes. However, following a visit to the hospital, I decided not to have the operation to remove the cataracts at that time. In 2005, I was told that I had an early bilateral posterior sub-capsular cataract and was advised by the consultant that I should not have the cataract operation yet.

Now I find that sitting too near to people I am talking to is not ideal because the vision field becomes so much smaller. I have to have a happy medium—I would say about one metre away. If I sit too close to the person that I am talking to, I will only see part of their face when trying to lip-read them. It is important that I see the expressions on their face in order to fully grasp their intended meaning. I really do rely on my hearing aids to help with communication and cannot manage without them, and, because of that, I need to face the person that I am talking to. I prefer to keep eye contact if possible and for the other person to keep their mouth clear of any obstructions.

TEN

Communication

Sign language is a visual way of communicating using hand gestures, facial expressions and body language. There are several different types of sign language used by deaf people for communicating with other people in the United Kingdom today. Here is a brief outline of British Sign Language (BSL), Sign Supported English (SSE) and Signed English (SE).

BSL is a visional means of communication that makes use of gestures, facial expressions, finger spelling, lip-reading and body language, and is the most widely used sign language in the United Kingdom today. It is not universal, and most countries have their own sign language, so British Sign Language is different from Irish Sign Language, French Sign Language or German Sign Language. In March 2003, after many years of campaigning, BSL was officially recognised by the British Government as a language in its own right. This was a major step forward as it paved the way to greater opportunities for deaf people in the United Kingdom. It includes the right for deaf children to be taught BSL in schools, the training of BSL and English interpreters and BSL tutors, a recognition of BSL as a valid academic qualification, and a greater use of BSL across society. Nowadays, BSL is used in many public places and can be seen on television, at theatres, in courts, and at public meetings and conferences to name just a few.

It is estimated that there are nine million people who are deaf or hard of hearing in the UK, but they are not all members of the Deaf Community. Deaf people who are members of the Deaf Community describe themselves as 'Deaf', written with a capital 'D' to emphasise their Deaf identity and they use BSL as their first or preferred language. However, it is estimated that there could be as many as 50,000 to 70,000 people who are BSL users. BSL, the language of the Deaf Community in the UK, has its own grammar structure, and it is not based on spoken English. For example, the question in English, 'What is your name?' becomes the sequence 'Name you what?' in BSL. The topic of the sentence, 'Name you', comes first, followed by the comment, 'what?' Here is another example, the question in English, 'Where do you live?' becomes the sequence 'Live you where?' in BSL. The topic is stated first, 'Live you' and then followed by the comment, 'Where?'

Sign Supported English (SSE) uses many BSL signs but uses the grammatical structure of spoken English, so different to BSL, which is a language in its own right. SSE is used to support spoken English, especially in schools where children have hearing impairments and are learning English grammar, or by people who mix mainly with hearing people. Secondly, some deaf people do not use BSL, but Sign Supported English (SSE). SSE is not a language in its own right like BSL, but more a kind of English with signs. Many people you see signing may be using SSE. Some people use neither SSE nor BSL but elements of both, so that their signing is somewhere in between the two. For this reason, it is hard to give an exact figure for the number of BSL users. Many people who are born deaf or become hearing impaired during their early life may sign to communicate with other people while hearing people may use BSL because they have family members or friends who are deaf. Children who have hearing parents may learn to sign when they meet other deaf children at a deaf school. Signed English (SE) is when every word is signed, in the correct English grammar order. This is for people who are only moderately deaf or severely deaf and do not want to use the BSL structure.

There are an estimated 23,000 people in the UK who are deaf/blind (sight and hearing impaired). There are several different ways that deaf/blind people can communicate with other people—by using speech, hearing aids, lip-reading, finger spelling, Deaf/Blind Manual Alphabet, Block and the British Sign Language to name just a few. The method used depends on how severe the condition is. Some deaf/blind people prefer to use tactile signing, such as the Deaf/Blind Manual Alphabet and Block, where words are spelt out on the individual's hand.

I did not find it hard being deaf when I was a little girl in the 1940s because I was never made aware that I was different from the other village children. It helped immensely that I had a strong relationship with my mother, however being deaf made me who and what I am—in fact, it is a massive part of me. I found connecting to the outside world to be very challenging, primarily because of the difficulties due to communication with hearing people being rather difficult.

The methods that I use for communication are speech, hearing aids and lip-reading but as my visual field narrows, it will become harder for me to lip-read. Still, despite attending two schools for the deaf, I never learned how to sign properly, which I now deeply regret, as I imagine that learning anything while a child is easier than when an adult. Some of my old school friends are experts, it would have been useful for me in everyday life, but would not affect my communication with my family, none of whom can sign, even though some have recently expressed the wish to learn. The manner in which people sign would have to change too because, as the field of vision narrows, the area used for signing would have to narrow as well. Many deaf/blind people find tactile signing, such as the British Sign Language and finger spelling, very useful. Although I admit that I am no expert when it comes to signing, I do know some signs and can do finger spelling, thus I suppose I will expand my knowledge in those areas as my need increases.

I am confident that I will always find a way to express myself. I am also aware that my limitations do not stem from the practical aspects of my disabilities, but also attitudes I encounter in the 'healthy world.' People should be aware of their positive or even negative feelings towards deaf, blind, or deaf/blind people, and try to make an effort to communicate with them. It is crucial to overcome fear, discomfort, or inadequacy, and possibly embarrassment that most people feel at first. These are some of the concerns of hearing people when I asked them about communication with deaf, blind and deaf/blind people. Some hearing people worry because they do not know how to start a conversation with someone who is deaf, blind, or deaf/blind and do not know how to help them if need be. I always ask my family and friends to touch or tap me on the shoulder or arm if they want my attention. Hearing people worry that they may be misunderstood and that this would put them in an embarrassing situation. This would only happen if they let it and if they are not sure how to approach a person with any disability, including those mentioned above, it is only because of a lack of knowledge.

Many deaf people wear hearing aids to hear speech and are generally excellent lip-readers. Some of my old school friends are totally deaf and can communicate well with hearing people. Can you imagine what it is like to live in a world of total silence? As many cannot hear their own voice and are unable to control it, they tend to shout or talk very loudly, and I agree that it takes a lot of understanding and patience.

Here is a bit of history! I cannot tell you who created the British Sign Language but I do know that Thomas Braidwood, a teacher from Edinburgh in Scotland, founded 'Braidwood Academy for the Deaf and Dumb' in 1760, which is acknowledged as the first school for the deaf in Britain. Thomas Braidwood's early use of sign language is now seen as the beginning of the sign language we use today. You might recall that, when I was a pupil at the Mary Hare Grammar School, I was in Braidwood House, which was rather poignant.

ELEVEN

Ronald took early redundancy

When Ronald took redundancy on 9th August 1990 because of his health problems, thus effectively retiring, he decided to become more involved in the domestic side of our lives. He offered to help me with the housework and shopping, but I preferred to do the work on my own as he would just keep getting in my way, but would be happy for him to help me with the shopping. Ronald needed a new interest to occupy his mind and I managed to persuade him to have driving lessons. Enthusiastic about that idea, he asked his doctor for advice and the doctor thought that learning to drive was a brilliant idea and even gave him the phone number of a driving instructor. Ronald made the call that night but the driving instructor was going away on holiday the next day and would not be available for three weeks. Looking back, it seemed odd that Ronald never learned to drive. However, as soon as our daughters, Anthea and Sharon were old enough to learn to drive, we paid for them to have driving lessons before buying them a second hand car. Anthea had a blue Ford Fiesta, while Sharon had a green Mini.

We did on occasion miss having our own means of transport, as was the case when I needed transport to get to Derby to attend a meeting that I told you about before. It took time for

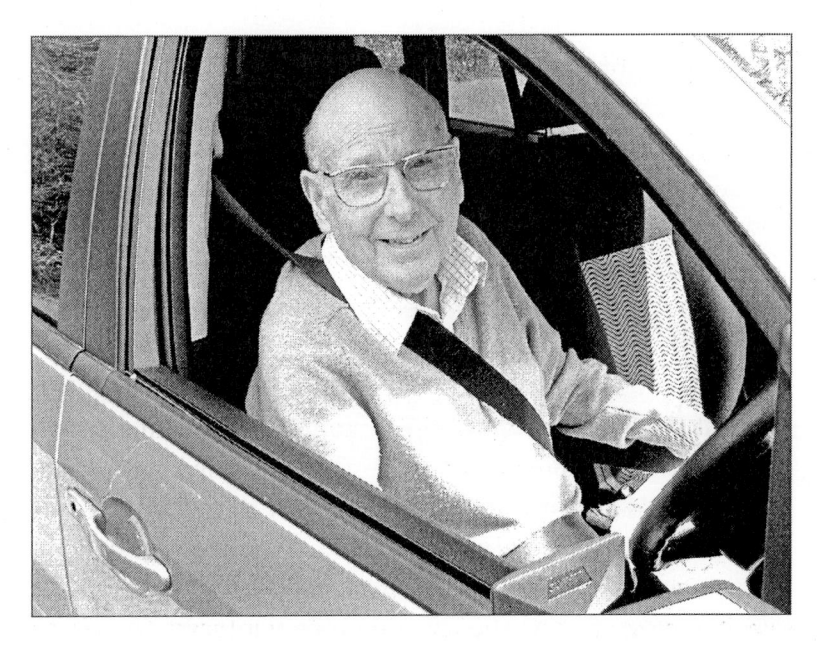

I have passed the driving test.

Ronald to think about it, as he was nervous about driving on the public roads. We soon sorted him out!

Coming back to the original story, with the instructor away, I did not want Ronald to have time to change his mind, so with the help of our eldest daughter, Anthea, we arranged for a relative who lived on a farming estate to take Ronald out for a drive in Anthea's car. Within a few days, Ronald was driving Anthea's car on the estate and enjoying it. As he found it hard having to change the gears, it was suggested that Ronald should use an automatic. Problem solved!

Some friends told us about the Motability scheme that enabled disabled people to exchange their Higher Rate Mobility Component of the Disability Living Allowance to obtain a new car. We went to GK Fords for more information and while we were there ordered a Ford Fiesta, but as Ronald had not passed his test at that time, we had our daughter, Anthea down as the main driver.

Two months later, Ronald passed his driving test at his first attempt at the age of sixty. To celebrate, we went away to Hunstanton in Norfolk for a few days. There was a rather funny incident while we were in Hunstanton, which I would like to share with you. Ronald had some shabby old white trainers that he liked to wear when driving because they were so comfortable. While we were in Hunstanton, we decided to go for a walk along the promenade because it was such a lovely warm evening. After parking the car, we made our way to the front and walked some distance along the promenade when Ronald realised that he had odd shoes on, one shabby white trainer and one ordinary black shoe, so guess what, he limped all the way back to the car, sometimes I really did not know what to think of him!

Having a car made it easier for us to get about, especially when going away on holiday. I will never forget the holiday with Ronald's sister, Pat and brother-in-law, Francis when we went to Coldingham in the Scottish Borders, as nearby was St Abbs, a quaint fishing village and St Abbs Nature Reserve. St Abbs is on the east coast of Scotland and serves as a centre for underwater diving due to its clear waters. We were lucky for as we arrived in the village so did two divers and they were sorting out all their gear and equipment and not only that, they practically gave us a running commentary!

We asked them questions about underwater diving and they were happy to tell us all about it. We watched them enter the water and disappear from view—unfortunately, we could not stay as we needed to move on so that we could carry on with the itinerary planned for the day.

To the north of the village is St Abbs Head Nature Reserve with a large colony of seabirds. We did not go too near the edge of the cliff as it was breeding time—June to July. The cliffs are inhabited by large colonies of guillemots, kittiwakes, fulmars and razorbills, to be honest I do not know which is which but it was marvellous to see the seabirds nesting and to be so near to them but they did make a lot of noise! We went on a boat trip too and I am so glad that we did for the trip was a wonderful experience. The coastline was stunning and seabirds that can be found there include kittiwakes, fulmars, guillemots, razorbills, shags and puffins. The coastline of cliffs and narrow gullies was really beautiful and we were so amazed at the number of seabirds flying around—there were thousands!

With my mobility made much easier by having our own car, I was much more positive. I try to be more organised, so that my disabilities would have very little effect on my daily life. For example, my hearing aids are always in the same place in front of my alarm clock, so that I know where they are should I need them during the night. I have been wearing hearing aids since I was about eight years old. The first one was an analogue hearing aid that I was fitted with when I became a pupil at the Maud Maxfield School in Sheffield. I've had several during my lifetime and now wear digital hearing aids.

Without my hearing aids, I would not be able to hear the everyday sounds that most hearing people would probably take for granted, such as the alarm clock, the click of the kettle when the water has boiled, bleeps on the microwave and the knock on the door. Yes, there are many challenges that I have to face, ranging from using the telephone and even watching the television. Thankfully, nowadays, there are many devices that can help to overcome these difficulties. I visit the websites of 'Action on Hearing Loss' (RNID) and the 'Royal National Institute for the Blind' (RNIB) and regularly look at their catalogues or visit their online shop to look at their problem solving products and I have found both organisations to be extremely helpful and useful.

I have an alarm clock that is not only rather loud, but also has a vibrating pad that is put under my pillow. When the alarm goes off, the pad vibrates and wakes me up, which is brilliant. A representative from the Deaf and Hearing Support demonstrated some doorbells at my home and I am delighted with the one I chose. It has an excellent door chime and a flashing blue light, both of which are activated when the push button on the front door is pressed.

A useful gadget that I purchased from the RNIB and one that I must mention is a liquid level indicator which hangs outside the container that I am going to fill. I use it especially when I am making a hot drink. The indicator will detect two levels of liquid. When I am pouring some tea into a cup and it is nearly full, I will feel a series of intermittent vibrations to warn me that the cup is nearly full. When the second level is detected by the indicator, a continuous vibration is given out and at that stage I stop pouring immediately. This gadget solved a problem as I had a tendency to over spill when pouring liquids into containers.

I also purchased a large button telephone with pictures, which I find very easy to use. The phone contains 'direct dial' buttons in which the full phone number of family members I contact regularly have been programmed. I have also inserted their photographs, so all I have to do is press the photograph of the person that I want to contact. The telephone has a volume control to increase or decrease the sound. However, as a hearing aid user, I find the 'T' setting optimal. Some of you may wonder what a 'T' setting is, so I will elaborate. When I turn on the 'T' setting on my hearing aid, it activates a very small device in the hearing aid that enables it to work with an induction loop or a telephone with an inductive coupler. I am then able to hear sounds more clearly with no interference from any background noise.

I find that hearing aids are getting more sophisticated and helpful all the time; my hearing aids are provided by the National Health Service (NHS) and have provided a lifeline. For example, I recall a rather poignant experience a few years ago, when Ronald and I were on holiday in the Yorkshire Dales. I heard a thrush singing, it was beautiful. I know that it is not possible for me to hear the sounds that people with normal hearing do but it was still beautiful. Ronald called me over to the large bedroom window at the Bed and Breakfast place where we were staying. It was a beautiful day and the windows were open, so he told me to sit by the window and listen carefully to the sounds of nature, that was when I heard the thrush singing. I was so excited, and I asked Ronald if he knew where the thrush was, he pointed it out to me. Some weeks before the holiday, I was fitted with two new digital hearing aids and I am sure that was the reason why I could hear the thrush singing. I will always treasure that moment. When I had my new digital hearing aids, I found that I could hear much more. There were many sounds that I did not recognise—sounds that I have never heard before or probably not noticed them. It took a while for my brain to recognise and remember what I was now hearing, such as the sounds of the birds singing.

What is it like to be hearing? I do not know, but I can imagine that some hearing people must sometimes wish that they were deaf! I do not mean it literally, but I have heard people say that they wished that they were deaf like me, especially when the children are making so much noise and driving them up the wall! Still, there are certainly some benefits to being deaf. For example, I did not wake up because my husband was snoring—when I was snoring, he woke up and then could not get to sleep again. I sleep through thunderstorms and no noise would disturb me. When people phone our home and ask if they can do a market survey, or explain that they would be in the neighbourhood in the near future and ask if they can call, or if we want some new windows or whatever, it is usually someone with a strong accent that I cannot follow or someone talking so fast that I do not understand anything they are saying—it sounds like one very long word. I start telling them that I am deaf and do not understand what they are talking about and they usually hang up on me, for which I am usually grateful. Still, there are many disadvantages, including listening to the radio or television and not being able to follow what is being said. Similarly, not being able to take part in a group conversation and trying to talk to someone when there is a lot of background noise, it is often challenging.

I have also learned to cope with my declining vision quality by coming up with some 'tricks' that I found on the RNIB website that I can use when trying to perform everyday tasks. For example, I have a colour-indicating button on most of my clothes to help me to identify the different coloured items. On a pair of black trousers, I have a black square button sewn on, while on a navy blue pair there is a navy eight point star button. This has proved an excellent idea. On some of our household equipment, such as the television, I have a red raised bump marking the on/off position—these "bumpons" are supplied on a self-adhesive backing and have proved very helpful in finding the on/off positions very quickly. Other useful items that I have purchased include "sokloks," which will ensure that I will never lose a sock in the wash again. My husband was very happy about that, as he had loads of odd socks and still kept hoping that the other socks would eventually turn up!

As I am not good with recognising different colours, I am not confident with buying new clothes, so I rely on shopping expeditions with Anthea and Lauren to Meadowhall in Sheffield to help me stock up on essentials. We always have lots of fun, even though I am certain that Anthea must have gotten exasperated with me at times. I go shopping with Sharon as well, on such occasions, she just gets a pile of clothes and we go to the fitting room where I try everything on—we have lots of fun! I find it difficult to recognise some colours, as to me they are so pale that they hardly register as a colour. I hate it when there is not much colour about as it makes things look so dull and drab. In particular, I am not keen on dark colours such as black, navy blue, brown and dark green as I find it very hard to distinguish between them.

I had good reading vision until my late middle age but, nowadays, I find reading hard work, rather than the pleasure that it once was. At one time, I enjoyed reading books, magazines and newspapers. Now, however, even though I do have gadgets to help me to read, the experience is not the same. When I told my rehabilitation support worker that I was having difficulty with reading my mail and was having to rely on my daughters, Anthea and Sharon, to sort things out for me, she suggested that she contact the Low Vision Aids Department at the local hospital and ask someone to show me the monomouse. 'A monomouse, whatever is that?' I am sure you are now asking—it is a handheld CCTV magnifier, a computer shaped mouse device that has an integral black and white video camera that can be linked via a scart connection to a television. When the mouse is connected to the television and placed on a document or text, the television displays a magnified image. By using this device, I am now able to read my mail, magazines and so on. It just goes to show that you should discuss your problems, as there is a good chance that there are some people that can help to solve them!

For people with disabilities, there will always be some problems to overcome, and for me some were reasonably easy to sort out, compared to others. For example, at mealtimes, Ronald would usually point out where different items are on the table, such as my glass of water, and he would pass the condiments over to me and anything else that I would need, rather than allow me to reach for them, as I am liable to knock things over. I also found that it was better to have a plain coloured tablecloth, such as a green one, rather than a colourful patterned or multi-coloured one. For tumblers or glasses, I found that it would be better if they were coloured or had a strong coloured pattern on them, though this is still no guarantee that I would not knock anything over.

One Christmas, when Ronald and I went to our daughter Anthea's home for Christmas dinner, instead of giving me a wine glass, Anthea gave me an attractive cup to drink out of during our lovely meal and I was very comfortable with that and did not knock it over. Little things such as asking my husband not to move things so that I know where they are do help, even though I find that, most of the time, I am the one moving things and furniture around!

Although I particularly love spending time with our daughters and grandchildren, I do have hobbies. I have always enjoyed sporting activities but nowadays my interest has moved to photography, family history, walking in the countryside, music and computers. I had my first camera in 1952; it was a folding Brownie camera. I still have it and will not part with it for sentimental reasons, as it was a gift from my mother and father. At present, I have a Canon Power Shot SX 200, which I believe to be a great little camera and I have been able to take some great images. Well, at least I think so!

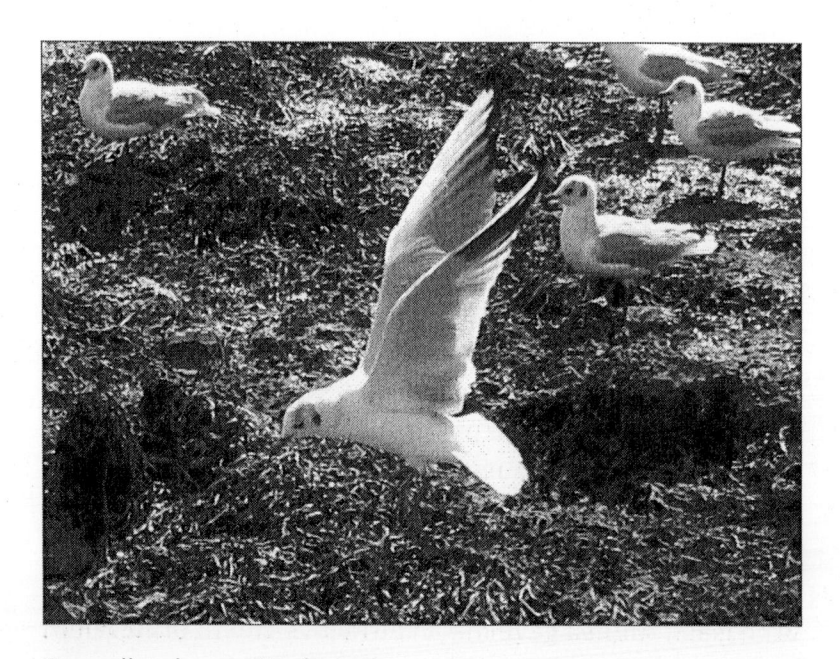

Seagull, taken at Keyhaven.

Sunset, Milford on Sea.

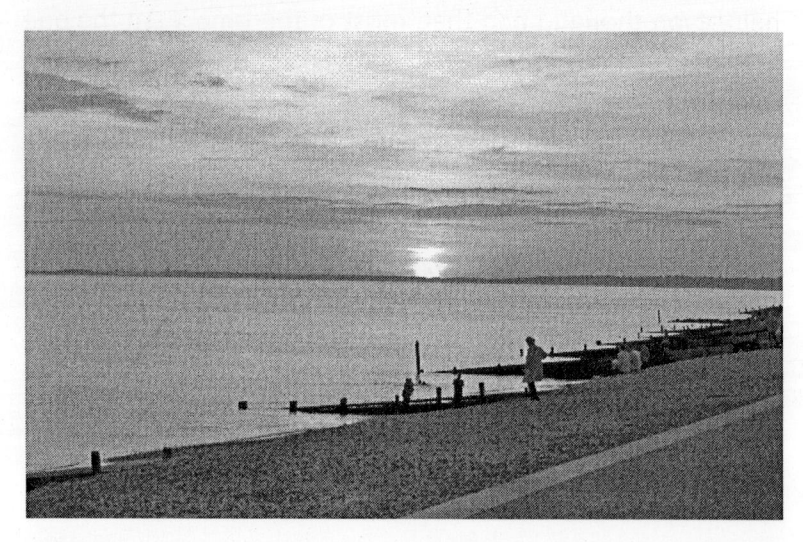

One summer, Ronald and I went to the New Forest with my stepsister Rosalyn and her husband, Paul. We all had our cameras with us and took lots of images. One lovely afternoon at Keyhaven, we were sitting on a bench, watching some gulls flying around; when I told Rosalyn that I wished that I could take some shots of the gulls but was unlikely to be quick enough. Paul called over that he had some cold chips in his bag and that he would throw them into the air so that I could take some shots of the gulls. My first attempt was a complete failure because I was not aiming my camera in the same direction as Paul was throwing the chips! We decided to have another go, this time making sure that we both knew what we had to do. When we were both ready, I held my camera up and using the wide angle lens took some shots of the gulls, By taking photographs using my wide angle lens and then using the 'trimming tool' on the camera, I created some fantastic photos. It helps to produce close-ups of birds, animals, flowers and many more—it is a very useful tool for people with vision problems.

As one of my other passions is learning more about my family, for a number of years now, I have been tracing my family history. In my search, I have been tackling archives, libraries, as well as asking for help from many organisations devoted to family history and trying to find my way around the increasing number of resources on the internet. Using the internet for research has been very useful, mainly because of the ability to get in touch with fellow researchers quickly and efficiently from my computer and others. I have exchanged information with researchers from Australia, New Zealand, Canada, Channel Islands, USA, Ireland and England to men-

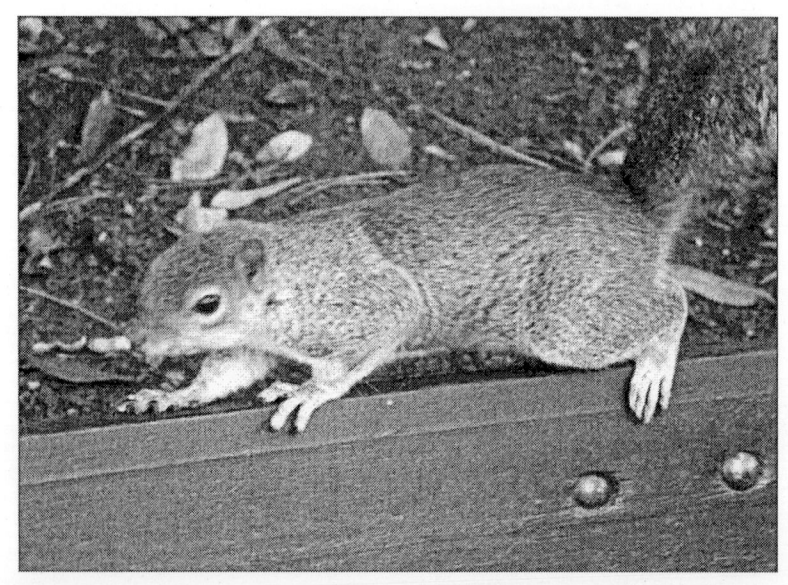

Grey squirrel, taken at the Winter Gardens in Bournemouth.

Seagull, taken at Milford on Sea.

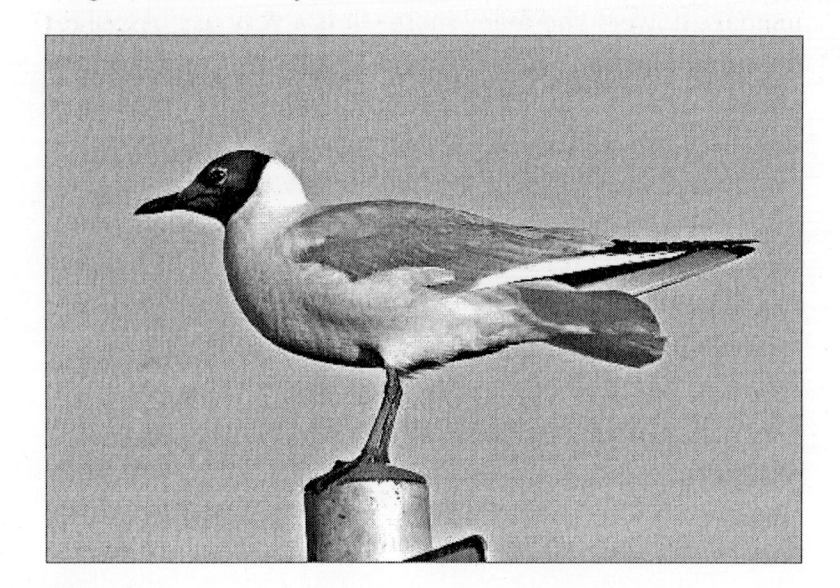

tion just a few. Ronald and I have also visited different Archives and Record Offices, and different churches, so that we could look at the headstones. In our pursuit, we sometimes ended up with strangers helping us. We had lots of fun and enjoyed meeting other people who had similar interests. We were also privileged to have the opportunity to talk to some of the vicars, who were very helpful. We got wet many times and ended up with muddy shoes, but we still had a great time. I have found lots of information regarding my family and my husband, Ronald's line and, as it is an on-going project, I am hoping that other family members will carry on with the work.

I enjoy sitting in a comfortable armchair, listening to music particularly from the musicals by Sir Andrew Lloyd Webber. A group of us went to see *The Sound of Music* starring Connie Fisher in London. I really enjoyed it and even though the light conditions made it difficult for me at times, it was fantastic. I have no particular favourite singer, as there are so many that I enjoy listening to, including Russell Watson, Susan Boyle, Lesley Garrett, Katharine Jenkins, Alfie Boe and Elaine Page. I do tend to have the music on too loud so have started to wear headphones which I find to be so much better. My husband, Ronald had similar tastes in music, but also tended to listen to classical music more.

I do not know what I would do without my computer—I enjoy surfing the web, researching my family history, being the administrator of our private family website and writing my two blogs on blogger. There is so much that you can do and it is a lovely way to keep in touch with family and friends.

As I enjoy taking photographs and downloading them on to my computer from my camera, I also have some fun editing them. There is so much that you can do with photographs these days, such as producing calendars, greeting cards and slideshows.

When my father and stepmother, Hilda, lived in Scarcliffe, Ronald and I visited them every week. Sadly, my father, George, lost Hilda in 1999 after a short illness and forty three years of married life. For many years, my father had not enjoyed good health. Ronald and I continued to visit him every week seeing to his needs. We also arranged for meals to be delivered to him and for a cleaner to come regularly, during the week, so that we knew that he was safe and cared for. One day, when he was eighty-eight years old, he was a victim of a burglary and a few weeks later he suffered a nasty fall at his home. He was admitted to a Care Centre to help him to recover, but it became obvious that he was not capable of looking after himself and needed to be in a home. Later, he was moved to a Care Home near Chesterfield, where our family home is, so that we could continue to visit him regularly.

I will always treasure the last few weeks of his life, as, due to his deteriorating health, he thought that I was his sister, even though, at that time, this would make me 93 years old—obviously a very young and energetic 93 years old! He smiled at me when I walked into the Care Home, held my hands and told other carers that his sister had come to see him. I was grateful when the staff agreed to my request not to correct him when he called me his sister. My father, George Elliott, died on 9th January 2006, aged 91.

TWELVE

Mobility

In some ways, my husband, Ronald had been my ears and eyes for years, as we always went out together and he helped me navigate around our home too. During our outings, he would point out things of interest and make sure that I did not stumble or bump into anything. Whenever Ronald pointed at something in the sky, I would moan at him and complain that, for me, it was like looking for a needle in a haystack, especially on a clear day. Still, he was determined for me not to miss out on anything and would usually insist on my having a look.

Sharon told my husband, Ronald and me that she loved the fact that we were still romantic after being married for a long time and that we should bottle our secret and make a fortune out of it! I smiled and asked her what she was talking about and she told us that whenever we were out we were always holding hands. I laughed and told Sharon that even though I loved holding her dad's hand it was more to guide me and keep me safe than it was about being romantic, Sharon looked disappointed! Ronald and I had developed a system over the years which meant that I did not always feel like I was being led everywhere and we could walk and talk like any other couple. It must have worked very well as many of our friends would comment on what a wonderfully 'in tune' couple we were. We never told our secret to anyone as it would have ruined the illusion, even though Ronald and I were romantic in our own way.

Due to ill health, Ronald has not been able to go out much, this made me realise just how much I depended on him. Due to the change in our circumstances, I found that I was lacking in confidence when there was a need to go out to the shops on my own. I understandably became very nervous and reluctant to go to the shops and started to rely on other people to go with me. I became nervous about crossing roads, could not see in bright sunlight and had problems with glare. It was a situation that I was not happy with and I knew that I needed to do something about it.

I decided to apply for some mobility help as I felt that it would allow me to gain some independence and regain my dignity. I asked Ronald and our daughters what their thoughts were regarding the possibility of applying for a guide dog, and they were delighted with the idea. I got in touch with the Guide Dogs for the Blind Association and, after several meetings with their representatives, found that a guide dog was a feasible option for me. At first, it was suggested that I have some training with the long white cane, but I refused without any hesitation. The idea really did not appeal to me, but I later changed my mind and about a month later started my training. I knew that I should be more independent and less dependent on other people for help, though I have been very lucky to have a friend who often went into town shopping with me. Even if I did not need any help, I still loved her company!

About two months into my training, I fell down the stairs at our home. I certainly would not recommend that anyone should try it, for I was in pain for months and lost many mobility training sessions. I really do not know why I fell, and I wondered later if I missed a step or possibly misjudged the stair width—I really do not know. While I was lying on the floor at the bottom of the stairs, the phone started ringing and I told Ronald to pick the phone up—it was our daughter, Sharon, who wanted to know if there was anything we wanted from the shop. Though Ronald was very upset he did manage to tell Sharon to come home—realising that there was something wrong, Sharon immediately hurried down to our home. When I told her what had happened she phoned the paramedics—I was so pleased to have Sharon there with us.

I asked our elder daughter, Anthea, to put a message on the private family website for me and this is what she wrote: 'Just letting you all know that though my mum will be fine, we have spent the day at A & E with her. This morning, mum decided to try for a career change as a stunt woman. She has fallen down the stairs at home—full length from top to bottom, doing a somersault on the way down. She knew that she had hurt her back, so she stayed very still until the ambulance arrived to take her to hospital. She has been incredibly lucky and has not broken anything, although she is incredibly sore and bruised. She was looked after very well and fitted with a neck brace, until she was x-rayed.

'Unfortunately, she enjoyed it in A & E so much that, when they discharged her and she was leaving, she promptly fainted and had to be re-admitted for a couple of hours until she felt ready to go home. She is back at home this evening and Dad is looking after her. Looking back, it could have been a lot worse if she had not acted on instinct during the fall and stayed still until the ambulance arrived! Mum asked me to let you all know. Get well soon, Mum XX.'

It was several months before I resumed my mobility training and was eager to get on with it. I started on my long cane training, but first did a refresher's course, which was to prove very useful and did help to improve my confidence. After that, it was the turn of the long cane. The first four sessions were held at Christchurch Community Hall in Chesterfield. I was shown how to utilize my residual vision with some scanning techniques, such as looking for some keys that had dropped on the floor and scanning a room to note what was there.

The purpose of the long white cane is to allow me to detect obstacles at ground level that could be hazardous, such as kerbs or cars parked on a path, even though it is against the law. This technique allows me to use my remaining vision to look ahead and from one side to the other, with only an occasional glance down. As one of the symptoms of my eye disease is a loss of peripheral vision, which is often called 'Tunnel vision', this shows what a good mobility tool the long white cane is for the visually impaired!

First, I practised walking with the long white cane in the hall, and then I tried it on the stairs. I was okay on the stairs and, as you will already know, there are different types of stairs, some have handrails, some have landings, and some even include turns. When a handrail is present, I have to put the hand that is nearest on the handrail, as my other hand works the cane. I rest the tip of the cane on the second step in front of me and, as I go down the stairs, the cane tip slides forward and drops down to the next step. When it stops dropping and maybe slides a bit, I know that I am two steps from the bottom. When going up, I follow the same basic principle, except that the cane won't 'slide and drop', thus, I hold the cane, gently keeping it upright. Then I lightly press the cane against the step and slide it up to the next step, keeping the cane ahead of me by two steps. When the cane reaches the top, as it has no step to press against, I will know that I have two steps left before reaching the top. To find out how wide the stairs are, I move the cane across from one side to the other and this will also tell me if there are any objects on the stairs.

Later, I practiced walking along a pavement, which I found very troublesome because of the poor condition of the pavement, my long cane kept finding the holes and getting trapped. Then, there was a car parked half way onto the pavement. On approaching a corner, I was told to pay attention to what clues were available, as it was a route that I would use regularly and it was essential for me to have clues that would serve as markers along the way. After sorting that out, I learned how to get round the corner. Before crossing the road, I had to listen for any traffic coming and determine which way they were travelling. I found this hard at first, but with practice, I learned that I was able to distinguish which way the traffic was travelling. However, if I could hear traffic coming and I was standing close to the kerb, drivers will most likely think that I am trying to cross the road and will probably stop and shout to me that it's okay to cross over. I have been told to say 'thank you' and then wave them on. When standing at the kerb, if I could not hear any traffic coming or see any traffic with the limited vision that I have, then I would cross the road; otherwise, I step back and wait a bit longer. After we practised crossing the road for a while, it was time to return home and this was when the problems started! I was facing the sun and could not see a thing, as unfortunately, the glare from the sun was causing my eyes to run. As a result, everything became blurred, making me feel disorientated. I was told to try to keep going, which I did, and eventually reached the shade. It left me feeling a bit insecure and lacking confidence but I intended to persevere with the training but did wonder what I had let myself in for!

When walking along with the long white cane, it would sometimes get trapped in a hole or a rough area, which would result in me getting a jab in my abdomen. I avoided this by holding the cane a little to the right of my body; I found it easier and was told that, as long as I was comfortable and confident, and that I could use it effectively, this technique would be satisfactory. After a couple of sessions, though, I was enjoying working with the long cane but I still had my reservations. I wondered if the long cane would be a hindrance when in busy places, if people would move out of the way and let me pass or simply trip over it. I was worried that they may not see me coming probably because they are busy talking on their mobile phone or they may be looking in a shop window and suddenly turn and trip over my cane.

The long white cane that I am using now has a roller tip attached to the end, which maintains contact with the ground as I walk along. This indicates changes in the surface, such as when I am walking on the pavement and I accidentally walk on to the grass verge. As a result, I will immediately notice the change in texture and then realise that I have walked off my path.

Eventually, I found that I was becoming more confident and was beginning to enjoy walking out with the long white cane. I never thought that I would ever say that! The long white cane is a very useful and effective mobility tool and, though I resisted at first learning how to use it, I am so pleased that my rehabilitation support worker quietly explained to me its advantages. There were some problems, though, as I found that there were times when I had difficulties in distinguishing between the green grass and dark or mid-grey pavements. So, I would sometimes end up walking on the grass, but was shown how to overcome even this problem.

Any journey that I take can be dangerous, for roads and streets can be hostile to anyone with sight and hearing loss. Pavements and roadworks have to be navigated, as well as cars parked on the pavements. Why do so many car owners park their cars partly or wholly on pavements? Parking cars on the pavements can obstruct and seriously inconvenience pedestrians, not to mention people with prams or pushchairs, wheelchair users, those with visual impairments and the elderly. I was out using my long white cane, near my home when I heard someone saying 'Excuse me, please,' I was not certain where the sound was coming from but soon realised that it was coming from behind, when a girl, aged about eight, literally flew pass me on her bike. I was so pleased that I did not stop and turn around or she could have knocked me over. Yes, youngsters on bikes can be dangerous, too! To be fair, I would not like youngsters to ride their bikes on the road, as that could be too dangerous, but the children should be told that they should stop when there are pedestrians about and allow them to walk past before proceeding.

There are times when I feel that I need some help in getting around, as it can be difficult when in unfamiliar places or in crowded shops. The obstacles in the street, such as placards and posts, that are difficult to see, or should I say that I don't always see, may also put me in danger of tripping or falling. I know where the obstacles in familiar places are and am confident being on my own, but when in unfamiliar places, I feel much safer when in company. To overcome these issues, during my mobility training, I was shown some more techniques that I found particularly useful. For instance, I hate it when someone grabs hold of my arm and insists on looking after me because they do not realise how difficult and uncomfortable it is for the person with a loss of vision to relax and allow others to guide them. They may struggle being in control of their movements when others are holding on to their arm in an uncomfortable manner or as if their lives depend on it. I have been shown what to do should I ever find myself in that situation again, and I am not telling you how because I regard that as my secret weapon!

Most of my family and friends just tell me that their arm is there should I need any help. Hence, if I have any difficulty, and I do need help, I ask them to let me hold on to their arm and then I place my hand just above their elbow. At one time,

I could walk perfectly well on my own, but as soon as I have someone walking alongside me I cannot always keep track of where they are and it does not help me if I keep having to look round for them as I would then become disorientated. I was able to deal with most of my problems, but if I needed help I did not hesitate to ask for it.

THIRTEEN

Change in Circumstances

My husband, Ronald, died on 26th April 2011. He was admitted to the hospital and, within minutes of being lifted onto the hospital bed, he suffered a cardiac arrest. I knew what was happening, but I could not move. I was rooted to the spot until a nurse grabbed my hand and took me to another room. Shortly, I was told that the medical staff had successfully resuscitated him, but Ronald died a few hours later. Our two daughters, Anthea and Sharon, were thankfully with me at the time. As we sat at his bedside, holding his hands and trying to comfort him, we were there for each other as he slipped peacefully away. I was devastated when he died, but the thought that he was not suffering anymore was a consolation because he had suffered so much.

Ronald was my eyes and ears and always made sure that I was safe when we were out together and in the home. Although I will miss him terribly and find my life much harder without his love and support, I am positive that I can cope with my difficulties. Still, I am aware that I will have to make some changes in the home to suit my requirements and needs. As a way of helping me to retain my independence and mobility, my eldest daughter, Anthea suggested that I should start to rearrange the furniture and get rid of some items that I no longer need in order to give me more floor space, thus making the rooms much safer for me. I thought about this very carefully and, though reluctant to make any changes at first, decided that was what I must do to make me safer in my home. It was important for me to be more aware of my surroundings and, as I contemplated what to keep, I was reminded of an exercise that I did at the Christchurch Community Hall. I was asked to stand in the doorway and scan the hall, noting where the doors, radiators, windows, hatch, stack of chairs and the magazine rack were. Following that, I was asked to shut my eyes and then describe where everything was. I decided to adopt this system in my home by scanning the room from a chosen position and then created a mental picture of all its contents and their locations. This helped me to decide what furniture I wanted to keep or not keep.

My daughter, Anthea also suggested that I have a small tray in each room where I could place oddments so that I knew where they were, rather than leave them around in different places and then having difficulties in looking for the items. It did not look tidy and I decided to buy some decorative boxes. Now, by allocating special places for them in each room, I know where they are.

I enjoy going to Anthea's home for an evening meal now and then because it means seeing my granddaughter Lauren as well as her mum, dad, and Barbara, Richard's mum. Anthea always gives me a white plate while the others have a dark plate. This is because my white plate shows up more on the dark surface of the peninsular unit. Some people will tell me where the food is on my plate using the 'Clock method' such as the potatoes are at 12.00, meat at 6.00 and vegetables at

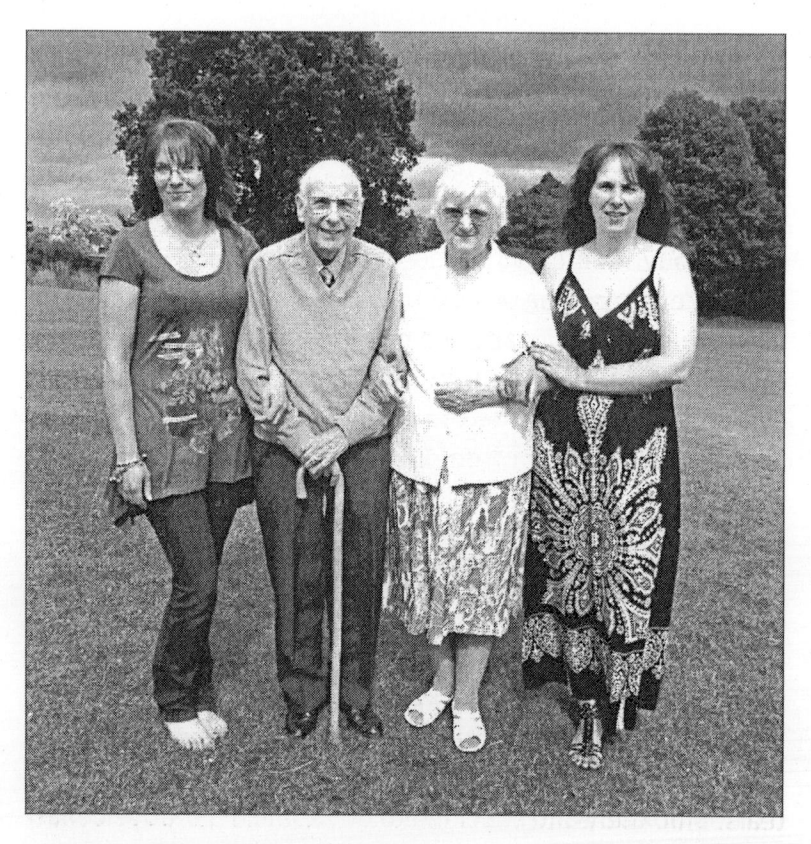

Anthea, Ronald, Jean and Sharon.

9.00 and if there is a Yorkshire pudding, I will be told that it is in the middle! Once, I was a bit confused because one friend sitting opposite me told me that my potatoes were at 6.00. meat at 12.00 and vegetables at 3.00 then I realised that they were looking at my plate upside down, so easily done!

Anthea gave me a very small torch that I have attached to my key ring; it is very useful for finding the key hole on the front door. It helps that I have a light above the front door and a wide step to stand on. I struggle to read the small print on food labels and packages so I keep a small magnifying glass in my handbag for when I go shopping. I have problems reading a menu when I go to a restaurant or café and have to ask one of my companions to read it to me—this could be one of my daughters or my stepsister, Rosalyn. In noisy places, it is not easy to hear what people are saying because of the background noise and the lighting is always low too, so now I usually ask if 'Jacket potato and salad' is on the list and if it is, I ask them to order that for me.

My youngest daughter, Sharon, and her best friend, Nicola decorated my living room and bedroom using contrasting colours that help me to note where the doors are more easily and I have found that very helpful. I love the colours that they suggested especially for my bedroom—raspberry and cream. I have been told that people with Retinitis pigmentosa are prone to problems with glare—this being the main reason for my problems at the moment and why I often shed tears. Still, there are ways of controlling glare such as avoiding reflective silk and gloss paint as these can exacerbate glare, hence why I asked Sharon to use matte paint. Most of the rooms have blinds so I am able to control the amount of light coming in especially on very bright days. When I am out on sunny bright days I wear some spectacles fitted with amber filters that eliminate the troublesome blue light while allowing the light needed for seeing to pass through. The filters also absorb 100% UVA and UVB. I have been advised to wear a hat but I am not what you would call a 'hat person' so I am reluctant to wear one but, I do wear a visor when it is really necessary.

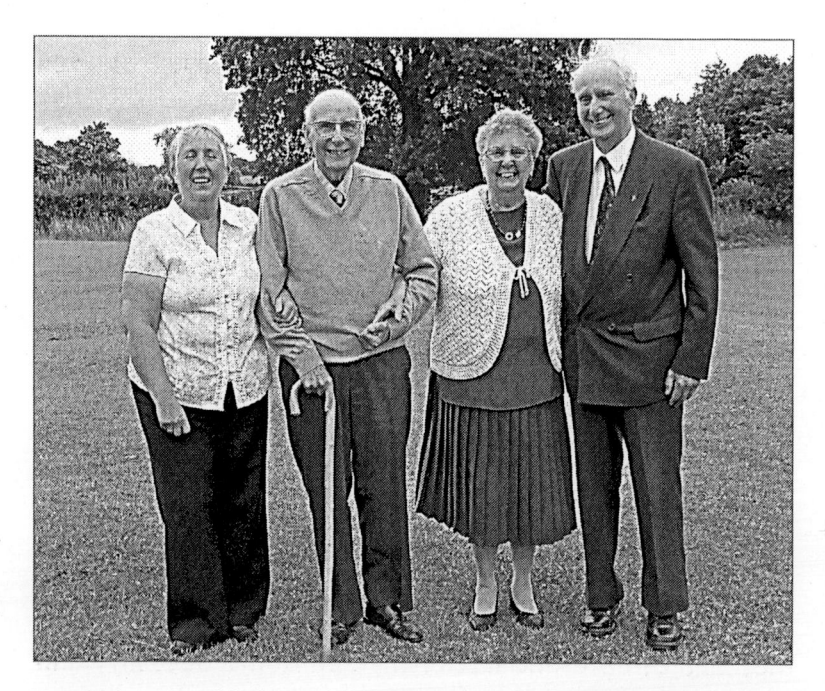

Ronald, second left, with his sisters Pat and Mary and his brother George.

I wondered what else I could improve and remembered the bathroom. In my bathroom, the toilet, toilet seat, cistern, shower cubicle, washbasin are all the same colour and the tiled walls and white ceiling did not make much of a contrast. I have increased the colour contrast by adding a coloured toilet seat and some coloured mats. On the wall is a lovely picture of some puffins hence, the new additions have improved the colour contrast making things more noticeable.

I went to a family birthday party and, during the evening, my sister-in-law passed a pile of birthday cards for me to look at. I kindly asked her to pass them on to someone else because everything would be slightly blurred to me. Her granddaughter, Emily, offered to show them to me and she read out the verses and told me who they were from as well as describing the card. It was lovely having one of the younger members of the family helping me! She was very patient and considerate. Her younger brother, Harry, came along after a while and told me about his new school and the football match he played in, scoring two goals. I am just as proud of my grandchildren, Jeanie and Joseph who come most days after school to see me and stay for about two hours doing their homework. Jeanie and Joe take it in turns to stay with me at the weekends too. I really enjoy their company and appreciated their understanding of my needs at such a young age.

My daughter, Sharon and her children gave me a lovely Mother's Day present—it was a Kindle Fire Tablet. My stepsister, Rosalyn showed me her Kindle Fire so that I could see if it was possible for me to use it to read e-books. I asked my brother in law, Paul to put a yellow background on and the largest print possible. Within minutes, I was amazed to find myself reading an e-book! I could not wait to tell Sharon about it and told her that I was going to buy one. Unknown to me, Sharon telephoned her Uncle Paul and asked him for information about the Kindle Fire and he gave her the details she needed. Sharon told me to wait until she could go shopping with me because there were several types and she wanted to make sure that I got the correct one.

On Mother's day, Sharon and my grandchildren came over for the day and I was given my present—a Kindle Fire Tablet! I gave it back to Sharon and asked her to set it up for

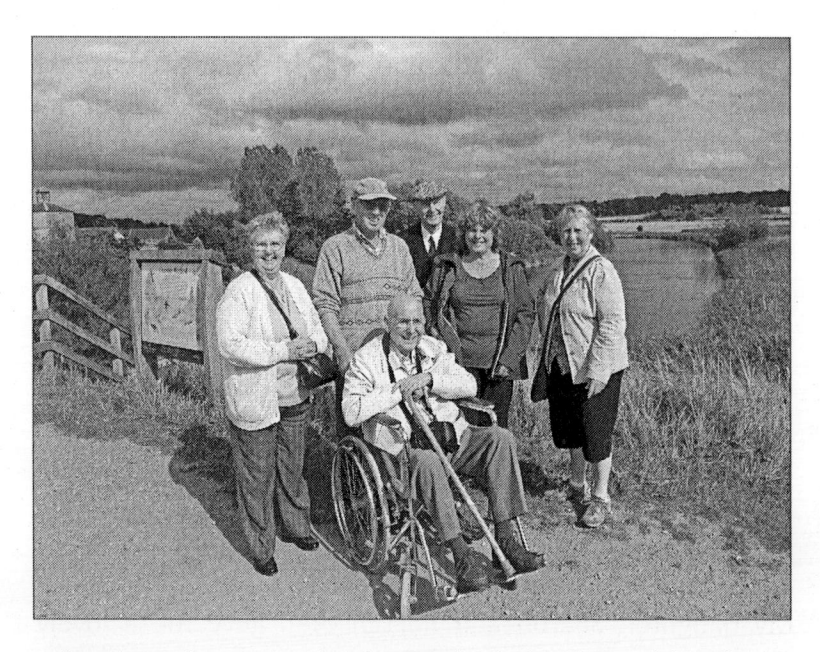

A family gathering in Clumber Park—behind Ronald in the wheelchair are, left to right: Mary Thelwell (Ronald's sister), Francis Buckley (Ronald's brother in law), George Reid (Ronald's brother), Teresa Solley (Ronald's neice) and Pat Buckley (Ronald's sister).

me. I found it much easier to read with a black background and white print which are the high contrast colours that I use on my computer. Eventually, Sharon asked me which book I wanted downloaded and I answered Rebecca by Daphne du Maurier. Changing pages with a touch screen was so easy but everything else I leave to Sharon! I have not had any problems reading the books on my Kindle Fire or with the tablet and I am so happy to be able to enjoy reading again.

What I want to do most is to do things that I enjoy such as spending some time with my two daughters, Anthea and Sharon and my grandchildren and going for walks in the countryside with Rosalyn, Paul and my guide dog, Ishka.

During summer 2012, I went camping with my daughter, Sharon and four grandchildren, to a camp site on the Isle of Wight. The site was placed in the ancient woodland on the outskirts of Ryde. It was a very peaceful and relaxing environment and we all loved it. There were some public footpaths and bridal paths that gave us access to the lovely surrounding countryside and coastline. When we were on the footpaths in the forest we would look out for the red squirrels—the only red squirrels that I saw were on some photographs taken by my granddaughter, Jeanie.

It took Sharon and some other campers who helped her, over two hours to put the tent up but as soon as we were organized we set off to Sandown where we had hired a beach hut for the week. During the evenings, Sharon and I would sit on our chairs outside the tent soaking up the atmosphere with a glass or two of wine while the grandchildren were having lots of fun down at the play area where they had made some new friends.

The facilities were fabulous—there was a disabled shower room with grab rails and a ramp from the path. All the shower rooms were brilliant, immaculate and just the right size to not get everything wet while having a shower. The main showers and toilets were spotless and the facilities for disabled people were spot on, but I did have a few problems mainly because of my limited vision. Whenever I went down to the amenities, Sharon or my granddaughter, Jeanie, would go with me but after a couple of days I felt confident with going on my own. I had picked a strange-looking tree to act as my marker where I knew that I had to turn right. The tree was my marker but, you guessed correctly, I missed the turning and the strange tree, and then I did not have a clue where I was! Still, unknown to me, my daughter, Sharon and the grandchildren were watching me walk down the path. Suddenly, the children kept popping up from nowhere and asking me if I was all right—I realised what was happening—they were trying to help me find the amenities! Eventually, I found the amenities and was then able to have a shower—they would not let me go on my own again as they did not want to lose their nanny!

At the start of the holiday we would buy buckets and spades, and beach balls and hire a beach hut. Sharon and I have always tried to choose a destination that had a beautiful beach as there is nothing better than spending the mornings playing with the children, building sand castles, and paddling in the sea. I will admit that I love paddling at the shore line and feeling the wet sand under my feet and the gentle sea breeze on my face. Sometimes I go in a bit farther and wait for the waves to break and splash over my feet. I could then feel my feet sinking into the sand which was gently creeping through between my toes. The children loved jumping over the waves as they break, squealing with laughter and shouting with joy—how they loved it.

During the night, I would wake Sharon up using an alerting device; it was actually a door-bell that could be used as an alerting device. I had the 'push button' and Sharon had the other end! If I wanted her during the night, I would press the 'push button' to alert her and then off we would go strolling down to the amenities in the dark—some tents had a light. I looked up at the dark sky but could not see any stars—I asked Sharon if she could see any stars, and she told me that the night sky looked beautiful. She asked me if I could see any stars, and I just shook my head and told her that the last time I saw any stars was when I was at the Mary Hare in the 1950s.

At the end of the holiday, we set off on a beautiful hot day to Cowes, to board the ferry to Southampton and then we travelled to Didcot in Oxfordshire where we had planned to stay for the night. The purpose of this was so that I could see Margaret who was my best friend when we were at the Mary Hare Grammar School and she still is. Unbeknownst to Sharon and the grandchildren, I'd been given permission by the Mary Hare School to take my daughter, Sharon, and the children for a walk around the school grounds and for Margaret to show them her Olympic torch.

We went to the Mary Hare School the following morning with Margaret leading the way—I had no idea of the route as it was nearly forty years since I last visited the school and it has changed so much. As we strolled around the school grounds, Margaret and I reminisced about the old days; we agreed that our school days were happy ones. Sharon and the children loved it, but you could see that they were a bit overwhelmed by everything. Eventually, it was time for us to depart and move on to Abingdon where Margaret lives. When we arrived at Margaret's home, having told Sharon that Margaret was going to show the children her Olympic torch, she told the children that Margaret had got something special to show them—her Olympic torch. The children were delighted especially when they all had their photograph taken holding the torch. After a lovely lunch, Margaret suggested that we all go to the park before setting off for home.

FOURTEEN

Charles Bonnet Syndrome CBS

Within a few weeks of losing my husband, I developed Charles Bonnet Syndrome (CBS), which is a condition that causes mentally healthy people with vision loss to have visual hallucinations. They were first described in 1760 by Charles Bonnet, a Swiss philosopher and writer, after noting that his elderly grandfather, who was nearly blind due to cataracts and cataract operations, had started experiencing visual hallucinations. He was being visited by visions of people, birds, carriages and buildings, all of which were invisible to everyone but him. It was in the 1930s that the phenomenon was named after Charles Bonnet in recognition of his work in showing that visual hallucinations secondary to eye disease are different from the hallucinations experienced by those with mental health problems.

I started to experience visual hallucinations at night when in bed and my first action was to hide under the bedclothes, well what else could I do? After a few seconds, I peeped out from under the bedclothes to find the stranger still there only to see him fade away. I can assure you that I was wide awake and I was not dreaming, but could not understand what was happening. I found this distressing at first and was reluctant to tell anyone—I decided to keep quiet about the people, children and patterns on the wall that I was seeing. It was really strange because what I was seeing was very vivid, detailed, colourful and clear, much clearer than the images I see in my everyday life. At this time, I was also struggling to cope with the loss of my husband. The hallucinations and the grief that I was experiencing made me feel that I had no time to be on my own with my thoughts and memories.

Eventually, when at Sharon's home, she commented that she was worried about me and wanted to know if I was all right. Sharon knew that I was struggling with the loss of Ronald, my husband, but she told me that I was quieter than usual. With tears in my eyes, I told her that I had a problem and did not really want to talk about it. Sharon told me that I could tell her anything and that she would always be there for me no matter what. After a few minutes, I started to tell Sharon about the people, children and patterns that I was seeing during the night and told her that it was usually about 3.00a.m. or 4.00a.m. before I went to bed. Thankfully, Sharon made it easier for me to deal with the problems that I was having because we were able to talk and laugh about what was happening to me. Still, I was quite reticent about telling people, but on a day out with my stepsister and brother-in-law I felt able to tell them about what was happening to me, they listened and made practical comments about what the problem might be. The next day I received an e-mail from my stepsister with a link to a newspaper article about a man who was experiencing the same night-time visions. She had gone home and searched on the internet and found the possible answer that I might be suffering from Charles Bonnet Syndrome.

Soon, I found that by blinking at the image, it would start to fade away, but switching on my bedside light would make the images fade much more quickly. I may get up and walk to the bathroom closing the door behind me, or stay in bed and try to concentrate on something else, or put my head under the covers and close my eyes. I knew that they were not real and that they would not hurt me, but could not comprehend what was happening to me or why. Eventually, I plucked up enough courage to see my General Practitioner who told me that there was no test available that could confirm that I had Charles Bonnet syndrome, but due to what I had told her she had no doubt that I did have the syndrome. Naturally, I wanted to know more about this phenomenon. My GP printed some information off the internet for me. Apparently, it can affect people at any age who have suffered serious sight loss, especially after a period of worsening sight.

The patterns that I see on the bedroom walls are mostly captivating, they are usually simple shapes and dots of colours, sometimes they consist of straight lines or of a mosaic pattern and cover all four walls and the ceiling. There was one pattern that I really could not make out but one night I could see it much more clearly, it was like a network of branches with flat leaves, as far as I was aware the branches and leaves were black and the background suggested that it was nightfall.

Charles Bonnet syndrome is a common condition that causes people who have lost a lot of sight to see things that are not really there. It depends too on how the brain reacts to this sight loss. When there is a lot of sight loss the brain does not receive sufficient information from the eyes as it did before.

As I have lost a lot of sight, my brain reacts by trying to compensate for the loss of peripheral vision by creating images to fill in the gaps. I have been told that the hallucinations may last for about a year, or it could be longer and then they will be less frequent but may not go away completely. One of the things I was pleased to hear was that these visual hallucinations do not indicate a mental health problem!

FIFTEEN

Living with Ushers

People with Usher syndrome want to live a life just like anyone else, but trying to fit in with a society that revolves around being able to hear and see can be very challenging—however, my aim in life has always been to lead an active life and to do the things that I enjoy the most. We all have to face enormous challenges in life and mine just happens to be a sensory loss of hearing and sight. The most challenging aspect is that it is not stable, and is a long lasting disease—I have had to adapt to less and less vision as the disease progresses and to how it has affected my life.

It is believed that sight and hearing give people at least ninety-five percent of the information regarding the world around them but, for a person with Usher syndrome, it will depend on how severe the condition is as to how much information will be gathered from the environment. Let me remind you of some of the most precious things in life that most of us take for granted—they are simple and ordinary, but precious. They are the five main senses—to hear, to see, to smell, to touch (feel), and to taste. Our five senses provide us with lots of information about our environment. Each sense plays an important role in our lives—the most effective way to receive this information is to use all our senses.

I have an inherited condition called Usher syndrome and during my teens started to experience changes in my sight. As the condition progressed I have had to face challenges adjusting to a life with a dual sensory loss of hearing and sight and having to cope with difficulties with communication, mobility, and access to information. Someone with a vision loss will most likely depend more on their hearing to compensate for a lack of visual clues from the environment. Similarly, someone with a hearing loss will depend on their vision to compensate for the lack of audio information. In people with a dual sensory loss of hearing and vision, neither of the two senses can effectively compensate for the lack of the other due to the impact they have on each other.

The information from the environment lets me know what is happening around me, such as cars and buses on the road, groups of people talking in the street, people waiting at the bus stop, children playing amongst themselves, dogs barking, and even a friendly neighbour when they shout out asking me 'Where are you off to this morning, Jean?'. I depend on my hearing aids when on the move to know what is happening around me and to know when it is safe to cross a road, but as my condition continues to get worse, there may well come a time when I will not know when it is safe to cross the road. It is vital for me to gather clues from the environment but, I know that I do not pick up all the clues by utilising my vision or depending on my hearing as both are impaired and so I cannot be certain that the information gathered is reliable.

My mobility skills have improved greatly since having my guide dog, Ishka, who was trained to walk in a straight line in the middle of the pavement, unless told differently by me, and to avoid obstacles along the way. Ishka will stop at kerbs and wait for a command to cross the road or to turn right or left. She will stop at steps, find doors and crossings for me and take me to places that we visit often—she will also guide me across the road but it is up to me to decide where and when to cross the road. Ishka and I are a partnership with me giving Ishka the commands, praise, and encouragement. We travel on public transport, explore the environment and go shopping.

When people with normal vision are looking straight ahead, they should be aware of movement to both sides. For people with Usher syndrome, this vision is considerably impaired, hence this is the reason why I bump into pedestrians and lamp posts, miss seeing overhanging branches, and trip over kerbs when walking outside. When I am indoors, I will often bump into furniture, doors, or cupboard doors that have not been closed properly. Looking for something that I have dropped on the floor and then having to get down on my knees to feel around for the lost object is bad enough! I use the scanning technique when looking for things dropped onto the floor—it amuses me and my family if they see me kneeling down on the floor, because straight away, they get down on the floor with me and then ask me what we are supposed to be looking for!

RP is a long-lasting disease that usually changes not by months but over many years. In the early stage, night-blindness was the main and only symptom that I had—in 1955 when I was fourteen, I realised that I could not see in the dark as well as my friends. Early signs of night-blindness may have been missed or ignored and being at a boarding school I was not likely to have many opportunities to be aware that I could not see too well outdoors at night. So the only problems that I had were hearing loss and the fact that I could not see in the dark, although I could see perfectly well in the day-time.

Having a dual sensory loss of hearing and sight does create many functional problems such as having difficulties seeing in the dark and I am certain that there are many people like me that try to avoid going out at night unless they have someone to go with them. I have to adapt between different lighting levels while people with normal vision will find that their vision adapts from light to darker conditions within a few seconds but for people with Usher syndrome, this adjustment may take several minutes, or even longer.

Walking around outside in dull or dark conditions can be very challenging; however, there are some precautions that I can take to help me. When leaving a brightly-lit place at night, it is advisable for me to give my eyes time to adjust to the new conditions. When I am out with my guide dog at night, I wear my fluorescent jacket that was provided by 'Guide Dogs,' as it is essential that road users and pedestrians can see me. I have got some fluorescent arm bands and belts similar to those that are worn by cyclists but I rarely use them preferring to use my jacket instead.

A guide dog is a mobility aid that can help people who are blind or partially blind to travel safely. My guide dog, Ishka, can guide me around obstacles such as wheelie bins and parked cars. She navigates through crowds in the town centre, stopping at kerbs, stairs, and steps. Sometimes she can even find a chair in a café or a seat on the bus—I just say to Ishka 'Find chair,' 'Find seat,' 'Find bus stop,' and 'Find door.' She keeps me safe when we are out exploring the environment, shopping in town, and when going to other places we visit.

Due to the loss of side vision, meaning the area surrounding my visual field, I do not see objects above, below, or to either side making it impossible for me to see objects unless they are directly in front of me causing me to bump or trip over things. This is commonly known as tunnel vision. There are simple things that are so easy for me to miss, such as not noticing a hand when someone offers to shake my hand, or when someone is offering me a sweet, or a biscuit on a plate. I bump or walk into various objects such as furniture, doors and cupboard doors. At first, I thought that I was just being clumsy—I did not know anything about tunnel vision until I joined the BRPS.

I am severely deaf and wear hearing aids—without them I would struggle to hear what people are saying to me. When I am having problems with understanding what someone is saying to me, I try to lip-read and watch their facial expressions and gestures for clues. However, communication is most important for me as I enjoy talking to people, watching the television, listening to music and the different sounds of the environment and would not like to be without my hearing aids.

I wear hearing aids, one in each ear and use assistive listening devices that have proved a lifeline for me. I can see and hear the television but I do sit close up to it. However, I do use an 'Echolink' when I am watching the television—this gadget amplifies the sound of my television and sends the sound directly to me via a neck loop so there is no need to have the television on too loud when I am on my own—I have to consider my neighbours too. It is wireless so there are no annoying and unsafe cables trailing everywhere. It always makes me smile when I ask people who have normal hearing if they can hear the television.

Recently, I purchased an Alto 2 from the RNIB shop, it reads to me with its built-in talking features. On-screen information is spoken and I am able to hear the button presses as well. When I scroll through my contact list I hear the names being read out and when I open a text message Alto 2 will read it out to me. Writing text messages is just as easy and as I type, each letter is read out aloud. It's also very easy to use with a simple menu and colour-coded buttons. I like the number keypad with the large and well-spaced buttons making it easier to hit the right button every time. I am pleased with it as now I can keep in contact with family and friends. I would like to have a smartphone, mainly so that I can download some apps that would help me with my daily life.

As for my reading, I am unable to read my mail, books, newspapers, and magazines but, as I have already explained, I have a monomouse. When the mouse is connected to the television and placed on a document or text, the television displays a magnified image. I go on the internet to read the *Daily Mail* and *Independent* as it is easy to enlarge the text size and I have a Kindle Fire that allows me to read ebooks.

Technology is advancing at a rapid speed today and is most likely the answer to solving many problems for people who have a dual sensory loss of hearing and sight. 'LookTel' is developing a suite of assistive smartphone applications to help people with low vision or blindness which will enable vision-impaired people to scan and instantly recognise objects such as packaged goods, money, and CDs —this would be brilliant!

SIXTEEN

Guide Dog Training

The Guide Dogs for the Blind Association, better known as 'Guide Dogs', is an amazing organisation, a charity founded in 1934. They have provided independence and freedom for thousands of blind and partially-sighted people by supplying guide dogs, mobility and other rehabilitation services. They also campaign passionately for the rights of those with visual impairments. It started in 1931 when two remarkable ladies, Muriel Crooke and Rosamund Bond, organised the training of the first four British guide dogs from a lock-up garage in Wallasey, Merseyside. The four guide dogs were called Judy, Flash, Folly and Meta.

After my successful match with Ishka, I could not wait to start my training at a residential hotel in Nottingham on 28th May 2012. I had been told that there would be two other people on the course with me—Simon from Doncaster and Kevin from Sheffield. I am delighted to say that we got on quite well—we encouraged and helped each other. Here is a brief summary of what we did on the course and you, too, will soon realise just how clever these guide dogs are.

Sharon and her friend, Nicola, took me to Nottingham with Sharon driving Nicola's car while Nicola did the navigating— I should have known better because Sharon always gets lost! While we were travelling down the motorway, Sharon suddenly asked me if it was Park Inn at Derby that we were heading for; I told her that it was Park Inn in Nottingham not Derby. We finally made it to Nottingham with about fifteen minutes to spare!

The first day was about orientation regarding the layout of the hotel. It looked relatively easy to navigate as the corridors were long and straight, lined with doors on both sides. Still, I did notice that in the area between the two fire doors there was not as much light as there was in the bottom half of the corridor which was much brighter. I navigated my way up and down the corridor by walking alongside the wall with my fingers or hand on it and feeling my way to my hotel room door by counting the doors as I walked by. My hotel room was at one end and the lounge was at the other end of the corridor on the opposite side, both between two fire doors. I was very surprised to find that I had difficulties in finding the lounge and my hotel room in what should have been an easy task—there were times when I got exasperated with myself. Still, with some help from my guide dog mobility instructor, I was eventually able to navigate my way around the corridor and only occasionally got it wrong—it was so much easier when I had Ishka to help me!

Later in the day, we attended our first talk in the lounge. The guide dog mobility instructor gave each of us a bag containing some equipment and asked us to empty the bag and she then told us what to feel for—the first thing that we had to feel for was the harness and then we were shown how to handle the harness. The harness fits round the dog's midsection and has a handle at the end which the owner holds on to. The handle allows the owner to receive tactile feedback and from the handle the owner can perceive what the guide dog is doing such as looking to the left or right or when she sits at a kerb or at the bottom of some steps.

Among other pieces of equipment were a lead which is used when walking with the dog when not in harness, in other words when it is not working. There were two collars, one of the collars had two bells on it and is regarded as a play collar. The second collar was for when the dog was working and finally a feeding whistle and grooming kit. This was followed by a discussion of the Guide Dog Agreement.

The second day, the day we had all been eagerly waiting for, was the day when Ishka, with whom I was successfully matched a few weeks before, was handed over to me. Before I was to meet Ishka, the other trainees and I were given a rundown of what to do on our first interaction with our chosen dog. We were told that there were to be no commands, just to be there and enjoy being with the dog. First, we had to make sure that our hotel room was dog proof by making sure that there was nothing on the floor or accessible to the dog—even the waste bin was moved to a safe place—on top of a table! I admit that I was slightly nervous or it could have been excitement while I was waiting, wondering how Ishka would react, but when the guide dog mobility instructor came in with Ishka, she dashed around the room sniffing at everything she could find. Ishka kept coming towards me and then moving away, eventually she decided to lie on her bed. I decided to sit down on the floor which proved to be a good move for she came over and sat near me and then sat alongside me. I did not make the first move—Ishka did by approaching me and sniffing around me. After a few minutes I decided that the time was right for me to make a fuss of her—it worked. After a short time on our own, the guide dog mobility instructor returned as it was time for the obedience training to start.

I did wonder if the real reason for staying at the Park Inn, a hotel in Nottingham, for two weeks was to enable the trainees to build a strong partnership with their newly-trained guide dog that they had been successfully matched with. I was very much aware that I had a problem, and that was the way I praised the guide dog—I am severely deaf and depend on my hearing aids, but praising a guide dog with my voice was proving to be a problem, and I have been told this repeatedly by people from Guide Dogs. I tried not to show it but the problem that I was having with praising the guide dog was worrying me.

My sister-in-law, Mary, suggested that I take her cuddly fox home to practise praising with it, and I did—took it home, I mean! One of Mary's friends sent me a small cuddly guide dog toy which became my lucky mascot. There were times when I felt that I would never have a guide dog, and, trust me, I did need one. I wanted a guide dog because I knew that it would give me the independence that I wanted so much, to be able to go out when I wanted instead of waiting for someone to be available.

To help build up a relationship with Ishka, I played with her a lot in my hotel room, made a fuss of her and talked to her—

yes, I knew she would not know what I was talking about, but it was better than ignoring her. It did not take me long to note that Ishka was highly trained and I can assure you that, as time went by, I was truly amazed at how clever she actually was.

There was an early start on the morning of the third day—5.30a.m.! This was so that the instructor could assist in the feeding of the dogs. After preparing the food I put the bowl down on the floor. Ishka, who was sitting nearby, started to eat her food as soon as I'd blown three short blasts on the feeding whistle—guide dogs are trained to do this from an early age. The feeding whistle is also used to recall the guide dog during a 'free run'—the dog has learned to link the feeding whistle with food; this encourages the guide dog to return to its owner knowing that it will receive a reward.

After the morning feed it was time to learn about grooming. Grooming is very important and helps to build a strong relationship between guide dog owner and guide dog. Ishka loves it when I rub my fingers through her coat against the lay of the hair. I would then brush her coat against the lay of the hair and then comb the coat in the direction of the growth. Finally, I would brush her coat in the direction of the hair growth. The job is accomplished after the equipment has been cleaned. This was followed by a mini health check and then by a working lunch when we were given a lecture about 'Dog Welfare' in the lounge.

Later in the afternoon, I went out in the van with the guide dog mobility instructor—it was only a short ride out but it was to an area where there was a small street block that was ideal for doing some harness practice. The commands that I used were mainly 'Forward' and 'Right' but the instructor did some work on my voice control as well! This is a weakness of mine, but the instructor kept on telling me to talk louder as Ishka could not hear me. 'Praise your dog, Jean,' the instructor would say! I tried—I really did, and I believe that was the day when I started to make some progress. I was beginning to feel more confident and only occasionally after that did the instructor find it necessary to remind me to praise my guide dog a bit louder—I was feeling a lot happier when I got my volume correct!

I went out with the guide dog mobility instructor and one of her colleagues on my own the next morning. Simon and Kevin and their dogs went earlier while I groomed Ishka in the lounge. The work this time involved corrections and swapping the lead from the harness to my right hand while walking with Ishka. Sounds easy enough, doesn't it—not to me, it wasn't! For some reason I was finding it almost impossible to swap the lead from the handle on the harness to my right hand while walking with Ishka. I admit that I did not feel comfortable with the lead between my forefinger and middle finger while holding the handle and it was noticeable that I was not holding the handle correctly—this was proving a big problem. I tried holding the handle and lead in a different way and although it was a slight improvement, it was not really satisfactory; however it was time to return to the hotel for lunch. We arrived late for lunch to find Simon and Kevin talking to the Fundraising Representative of Guide Dogs. Simon and Kevin went off with the guide dog mobility instructor to do some more training. I had an interesting conversation with the Fundraising Representative about the work that they do and told her that I would join the fundraising group in my hometown. After lunch, I did some obedience work with Ishka.

Later in the afternoon, the instructor asked me if I wanted to go out again, and my answer was a definite 'yes.' It was essential to sort out my difficulties with the harness and lead. The instructor showed me a different way to hold the handle with the lead and all of a sudden the problems were quickly solved—it was more comfortable and much easier for me to transfer the lead from the handle on the harness to my right hand by using this new method. By holding the handle, I receive tactile information letting me know what Ishka is doing and whenever necessary I can then correct her in the appropriate manner.

The next day, after doing our morning chores with the dogs, Simon and I met our instructor at the van and headed out for a training session at the Nottinghamshire Kennels. After arriving at our destination, it was suggested that I would go first while Simon remained at the van to groom Ascot. Our instructor had set up a course that had many obstacles enroute; it looked very interesting! There were lots of cones and other obstructions blocking our way, but not completely. We walked to the other end and then Ishka and I tackled the course—we did the course about three times in all. Eventually, we returned to the van while Simon and his guide dog, Ascot had their session. I groomed Ishka using the platform at the back of the van.

We returned to the hotel for a light lunch which was followed by a meeting with our District Client Representative who explained that if we had any problems she was the one that we should contact so that she could sort it out for us. It was a very interesting meeting and being a guide dog owner herself, she was able to tell us some funny stories!

For the afternoon session, Simon and I went out with the instructor to a small area where wheelie bins were littered all over the pavements! Simon went first and it was not long before he came back. I was looking forward to this exercise as this was obviously the follow-up to the obstacle course that we did that morning. Ishka and I started well, but it was not long before I walked into a wheelie bin and grabbed hold of it before it tipped over. The instructor told me that I should have let the wheelie bin go over, but I replied, 'No way, I am not going to end up putting the rubbish back in the bin.' The real reason why I walked into the wheelie bin was because I did not follow Ishka when she moved out towards the kerb however the instructor and I had a good laugh about it.

The next day, Simon and I had a very wet trip out—we went to a local street to test our skills of indenting. Simon went with the guide dog mobility instructor first while I stayed in the van. It was not long before Simon and the instructor returned to the van and then it was my turn. We set off and, to be honest, I did not think that Ishka and I were doing too badly in the very wet conditions but then it happened—I fell in marvellous style! Even though I hurt my right knee I wanted to carry on but I could not stop laughing. Eventually, the instructor and I returned to the van. The knee was sore for a few days, but I did not want to miss any of the training so I persevered with the pain—taking some pain-killers did the trick. In the afternoon, we headed to the hotel basement and did some obedience work. This work was done in front of the other dogs and this added numerous distractions but all the dogs did well—it was a bit too dark in the basement for me.

The next morning, after spending the dogs—taking the guide dogs to their pen to do their business—we all met at the van and with the trainer at the wheel we set off to a location nearby—it looked a nice area. I went out with the trainer first and, after a short walk, we arrived at some shops and I noted that one of them was a café. We went into the café and found an empty table near the window. Ishka immediately disappeared under the chairs. Oh yes, I wondered how many cafés Ishka has been in because you could see that she was no novice and knew exactly what she had to do. The trainer went to get me a fruit drink and then told me that she was going to fetch Simon and his guide dog, Ascot.

Ishka attracted a lot of attention from the other customers who asked if they could stroke her while others asked me what it was like having a guide dog. I explained that it was early days for me to answer that question as I was on a guide dog training course—throughout all this, Ishka behaved impeccably and I was really proud of her. It was not long before Simon and Ascot arrived and, after bringing a drink over for Simon, the trainer set off to fetch Kevin and his guide dog, Danny. Once again, some of the customers started to come over, again asking if they could stroke the guide dogs.

Eventually, Kevin and Danny arrived and now it was time for Ishka and me to depart—we walked along the street and eventually arrived back at the van—I really enjoyed that walk as it was a lovely day. When the others arrived back, we returned to the hotel for a light lunch.

In the afternoon we did some off-kerb obstacle training. This is when a guide dog cannot get their owner safely round an obstruction while on the pavement and so it means going onto the road, which could be dangerous for the guide dog owner and guide dog. Situations like this could happen when there are some road works, or a car parked on a pavement, or a group of wheelie bins standing close together. The trainer had set up some barriers which forced the guide dog to take their owner onto the road. This sort of thing happens a lot, especially when it is wheelie-bin day. Ishka and I often come across a group of wheelie bins standing close together and a car parked on the pavement, forcing Ishka to take me on to the road. Monday is our collection day and the day when we practice avoiding bins!

I am not likely to forget these traffic sessions! The idea was to get Ishka to move off a kerb while a car is approaching. I had to give Ishka the command to set off which I was not exactly happy with, for if anything went wrong, I would never forgive myself. This was how it was done—in a controlled situation with a colleague driving a car while my guide dog mobility instructor worked with Ishka and me. Imagine the main road being on the right and a car waiting to travel down the side road to join the main road. Ishka and I are waiting to cross the side street so the car will be on the far side and so we could be in the middle of the side street by the time the car arrived.

My instructor walked to the middle of the road and gave the driver of the car the signal to proceed and then came over to Ishka and me. When appropriately tapped on my shoulder I gave Ishka the forward command to proceed—we did this several times and Ishka hardly moved from the kerb because a car was approaching. We were just going to start the second stage when it started raining, thundering and lightening—Ishka made a dash but I held tightly on to her lead. We returned to the van very wet but laughing! I was very impressed with how Ishka reacted in the traffic session.

The night walk with Ishka was the last night, something that I was not looking forward to! The thought of walking around in the dark in unfamiliar surroundings made me feel nervous, as being in the dark is when I see the least. Having a dual disability is not easy—I know that I am unable to collect all the important clues from my surroundings with my remaining vision, and it is not possible for me to rely entirely on my hearing even though I wear hearing aids. I know—you must trust the guide dog, but it was not Ishka that I did not trust—it was me! It was simply a fear of being in the dark—I have not been out in the dark on my own for at least forty years. To be honest, I rarely go out at night unless I am with someone who has a car.

Kevin went out first and, as I sat in the van, I admitted to Simon that I was nervous, but I was going to do the night walk as I hoped that it would conquer my fears of going out in the

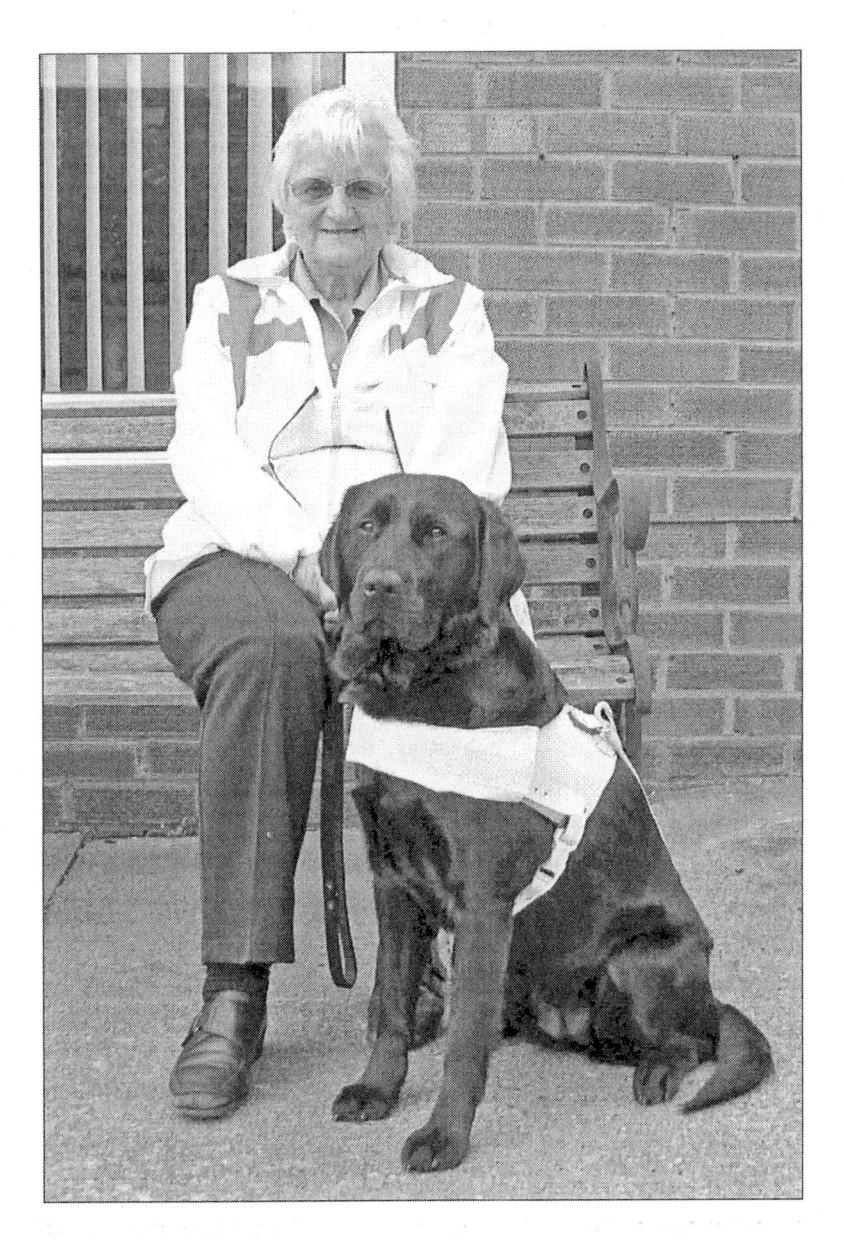

Jean and Ishka on the day that they qualified.

dark. Simon went next and then it was my turn. The instructor came round to my door and asked if I was ready and I replied that I was. We went round to the back of the van to get Ishka out—that was the first hurdle for I could not see her, but she came up to me when I called her name. I put her harness on and then it was time to go. We did the walk with the instructor talking to me as we went along and I trying to praise Ishka who walked slowly en-route, and then it was all over. Ishka was brilliant, and I cannot thank the instructor enough for her encouragement and understanding—I was pleased that it was all over.

About four months later, I did a night walk on my own, this time in familiar surroundings. I was not so nervous this time as I thought that there would be fewer distractions, less noise, vehicles, and people about and it was a route that Ishka and I knew so well—I had decided to go up to the supermarket and back. The first part of the journey was quite good, even though there were some very dark areas, and we arrived at the supermarket safely. I was very surprised to see how many people were there, some with their dogs, too, but most of the people were at the fish and chip shop! There were too many distractions during the second part of the journey, mainly because of dogs barking as we walked past houses but we arrived back home safely.

The last day of the course was when we had the 'free run' in a small enclosed field and it was great to watch the dogs chasing each other around the field as we walked slowly round with the guide dog instructor. This was an opportunity for us to test the 'recall' by blowing three times on our feeding whistle. The dogs came back running towards us as they knew that they were going to get a treat.

Following this, we all got in the van and our guide dog mobility instructor took us all home, dropping Simon off first, then Kevin and finally me. I was happy to be home again, but realised that there was still a lot of hard work to be done by Ishka and me—we did four weeks of intense work together before we qualified together on the 26th June 2012. Ishka was brilliant and made it so easy for me—I was so proud of her.

SEVENTEEN

Ishka, my guide dog

My life was much harder without Ronald's love and support, because of my difficulties in adjusting to the immense changes that were happening in my life at this particular time. I was suffering from depression, and started to withdraw into myself as I bottled up what was happening to me when I developed Charles Bonnet syndrome. I did not want to go out unless someone came with me, I was nervous crossing roads, going into shops and was increasingly losing my confidence.

Ishka in her favourite place.

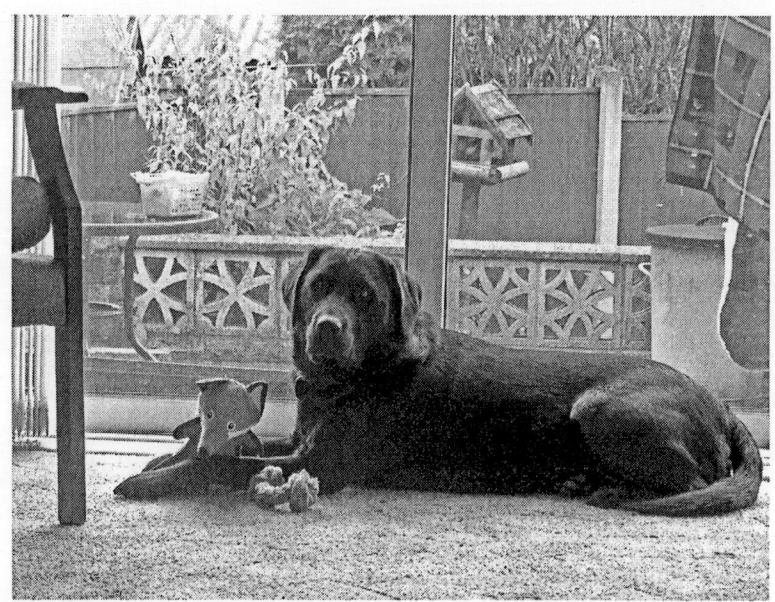

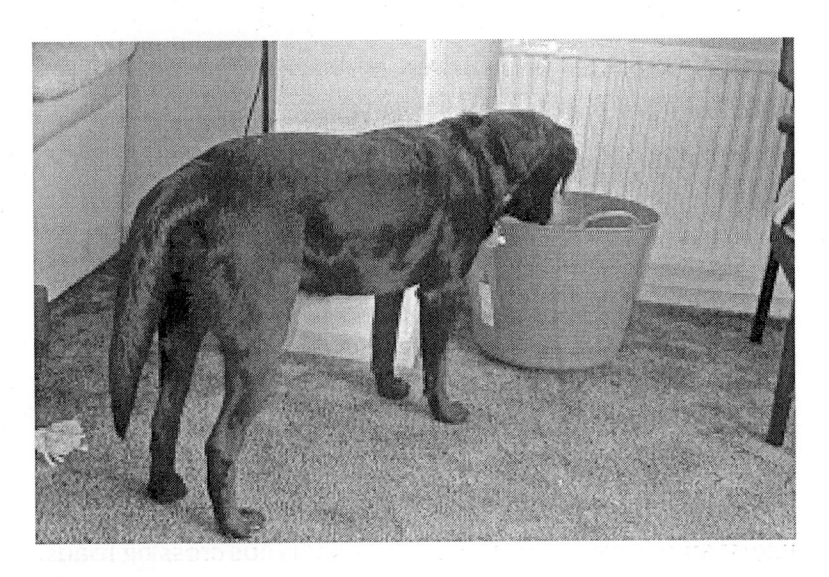

Ishka choosing a toy.

Since I qualified as a guide dog owner and Ishka as a guide dog on the 26th June 2012, a whole new world has opened up for me—Ishka accompanies me wherever I go, we explore the environment, go shopping, visit friends and relatives and go for leisurely walks—she loves going to Holmebrook Valley Country Park. We travel on public transport, but I have not been on a train with her yet, but will do so one day. Ishka has given me the freedom to go out to different places on my own and she has given me back my confidence, dignity, and zest for life. My life with Ishka is so much better now; I have only had one fall since we have been together and that was my fault.

I am a member of the Guide Dogs Fundraising group in Chesterfield and attend monthly meetings at the Rose and Crown in Brampton and help out with collections. I am also a member of the 'Deaf and Hearing Support' Board. The aim of this organisation is to provide free information and to demonstrate equipment to hearing-impaired people whose lives can be improved so that they will feel more included in society. Deaf and Hearing Support complement the services supplied by the Chesterfield Royal Audiology Department and Derbyshire Council Social Care Services.

My adorable black Labrador/golden retriever cross with a cold wet nose and a tail that is always wagging works hard in demanding situations. Our safety depends on our team-work and her concentrating when she is in the working mode—this is why people should not distract her when she is working by stroking her or by trying to give her some food. I am pleased that most people ask me first if they can stroke Ishka. I can tell her to take me to the bus stop, to PC World, the bank, the park, and other places but, most importantly, to take me home. There is now no need to worry about obstacles because I have got Ishka who will guide me round them—I have not walked into a post or anything similar for months! Ishka is my best friend, and when I talk to her, people laugh as she cocks her head to one side and then the other—she makes me laugh at her antics and is very playful—I am not lonely anymore. She gets very excited when meeting people she knows, but soon settles down again. She loves it when the grandchildren visit or call round when on their way home from school.

Talking about PC World, whenever we come out of the shop Ishka always turns right and takes me to another shop farther down—the 'Pets At Home' store. Once inside Ishka knows exactly where she needs to be—at the toy section. On one occasion while Sharon, my daughter, was with me, we were

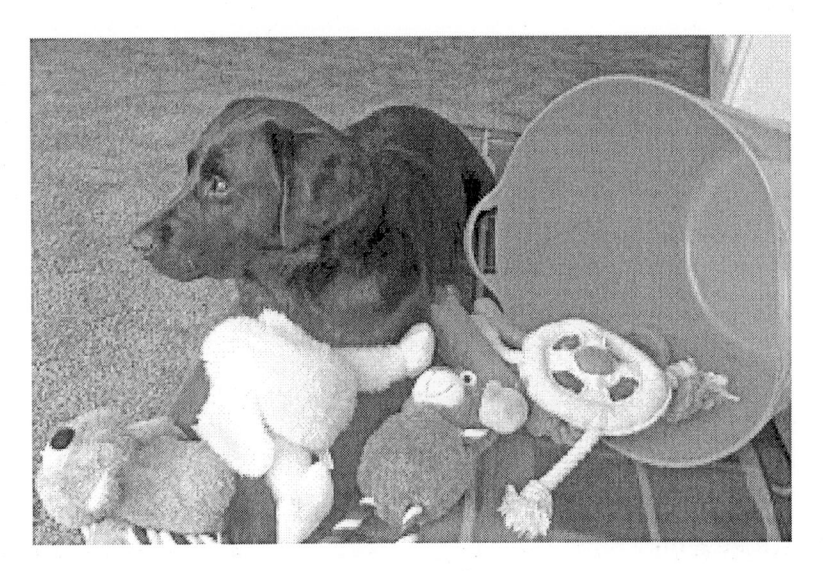

All my toys?

looking at the toys and Sharon heard some people laughing behind us. We soon discovered why! Ishka was holding a toy in her mouth looking up at me as if to tell me that she had found what she wanted and that it was time to go and pay—I have found that she has a liking for squeaky geese and now has quite a collection of different coloured ones.

Here is another story—a few weeks before Christmas 2012, we went into town to do some shopping with a friend. I told my friend, Barbara, that I wanted to catch the 4.30p.m. bus home before it got too dark, as you know one of the symptoms of RP is night-blindness. When we had finished our shopping and because it was very cold, we decided to go to a café for a coffee and cake. Unfortunately, we missed the 4.30p.m. bus and had to wait half an hour for the next one to arrive and by then it was beginning to go dark. We got on

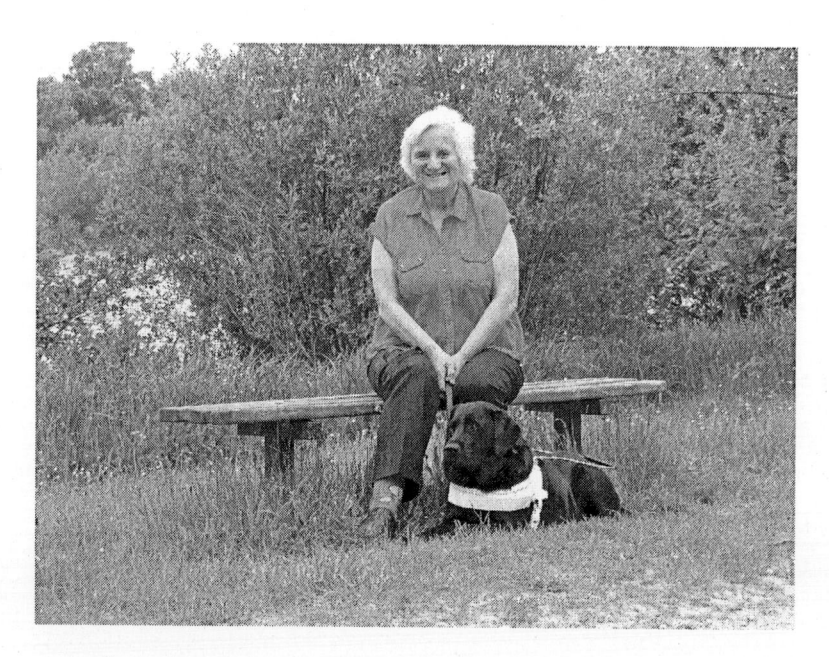

A walk in the park.

the bus and my friend got off a few stops before I did and by then it was really dark. Clues told me when it was time for me to ring the bell but the driver did not stop straight away—he carried on and went past the bus stop. When I got off the bus and the bus moved away, I did not know where I was as it was very dark and I could hardly see a thing. I turned toward Ishka and said 'Ishka, please take me home, take me home'. She took me across two roads and not long after, we arrived home to find my oldest grandson, Joseph waiting.

Ishka loves picking up socks and hankies—not just clean ones but dirty ones, too, and sometimes I will find the odd slipper or shoe in her box! I like to keep my kitchen door fully open so I use a door stopper but Ishka has found a way of removing the door stopper and that always ends up in her box too—mind you, I have not seen it for a couple of months! She wakes me up at about 5.30a.m. every morning and if I do not get up straight away, will try to pull my duvet off the bed but she has never managed to get it off. She loves to lie by my feet when I am watching the television—I did not think that she would enjoy watching programs such as *Emmerdale* and *Coronation Street*! She is always by my side and we play games with her toys. She loves to curl up by my feet and go to sleep, and when I fall down, which is very rare these days, she is there straight away as if to comfort me. What more can I ask for!

APPENDIX ONE

Ishka by her puppy walker, Julie

I had a dear friend whose eyesight was poor and who never walked past a guide dog collection box without first putting some money in, just in case she ever needed a guide dog one day. It was not to be, because sadly, she died at an early age. It was because of my friend that I took on a puppy from 'Guide Dogs' even though I have never had a dog before. We have lots of happy memories of Ishka from the day she ar-

Ishka at seven weeks old.

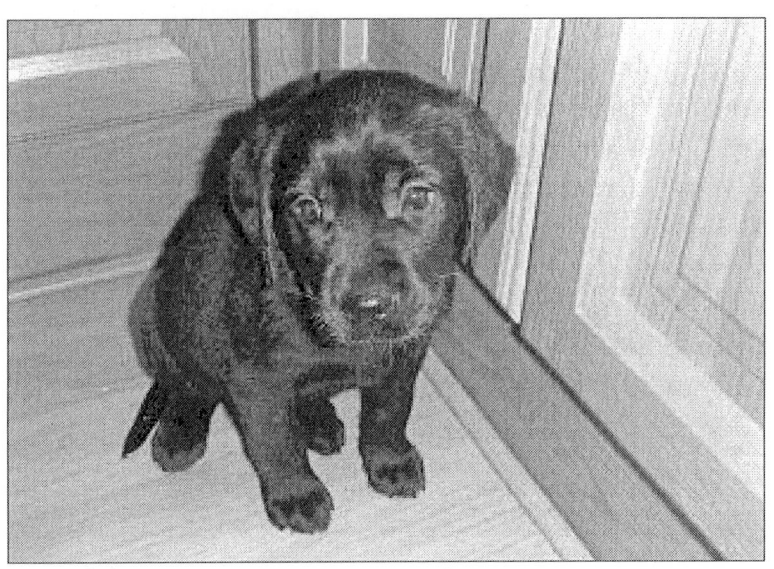

rived at our home to the last time that we saw her in Nottingham with her trainer.

Ishka arrived at our home when she was seven weeks old and as we watched her emerge from the transporting box, we saw a little black bundle of energy coming out and wagging her tail. We fell in love with her straight away. On the day of her arrival, Ishka weighed just 3kg. Her first bed was a vegetable box with a pillow to lie on and a borrowed fluffy vet bed blanket. Ishka's guide dog supervisor came along with a crocheted blanket for her to lie on when visiting cafes—these blankets are made by volunteers for all new puppies. At seven weeks old, Ishka was too young to walk outside so until she'd had her vaccinations I carried her safe and snug in a holdall when I went shopping and on the buses.

We praised, loved and introduced Ishka to different sights, sounds, and smells of her new world. We took Ishka shopping with us, travelled on buses, in cars, on trains, and walked along busy streets and she learned simple commands such as 'sit,' 'come,' 'down,' and 'stay.' Once there was an incident at Crewe Railway Station. We were trying to get Ishka off the train one evening when the heavens suddenly opened; it was a total nightmare! No matter what we did we could not get Ishka off the train. Eventually I managed to persuade Ishka to get off just before the train was due to leave the station. I really thought that we would be staying in Crewe for the night instead of Hartford!

Whilst Ishka was with us we went over to the Isle of Man, and stayed at my parents' home in Ramsey for three weeks

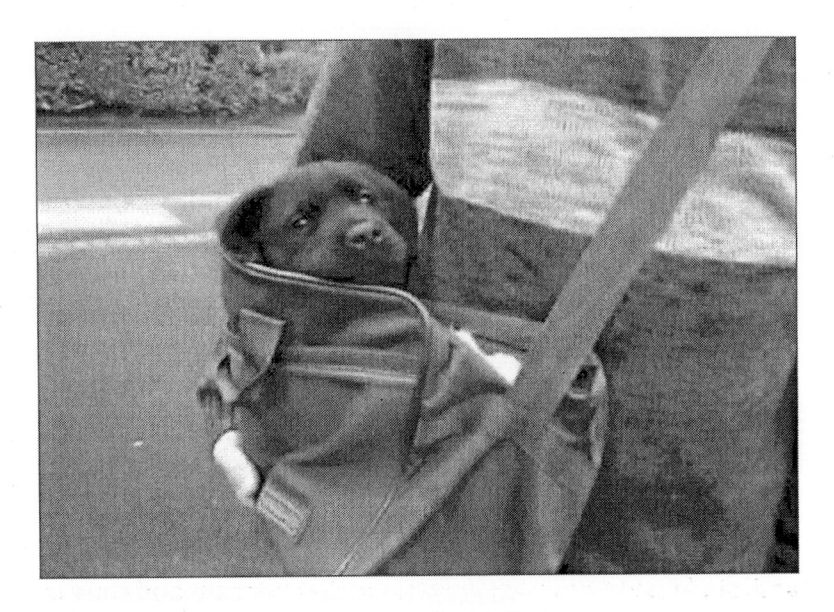

Ishka being carried around in a holdall

whilst I helped care for my mum who was recovering from an operation. Ishka had a great time as there were plenty of lovely walks in Ramsey and a wonderful beach for her to play on. The feel of the sand and stones beneath her feet was so exciting for her, but as for the sea and waves, she was not interested. Once there was an old smelly dogfish that had been washed up on the beach and this was far more interesting! She looked at us as if to say, 'Catch me if you can'. When I did manage to get the dogfish from her, it was to find that her breath smelled and it smelled for days, ugh! We travelled over to the Isle of Man in my car, via the Seacat—Manannan from Liverpool. It took two and a half hours so we left Ishka in the back of the car. She was absolutely brilliant and slept the whole journey—fortunately for all of us it was a smooth crossing. Ishka loves running into freshwater streams. We would throw a small pebble into a shallow running stream and Ishka would try to find the pebble. She really enjoyed this and would play until we were exhausted!

Ishka really likes soft toys and she never had a soft rabbit before so that is great that Jean, her owner, has got one for her. When she left us in December, we sent her to Atherton with a pink teddy bear called 'Chopsticks'. This ridiculous name was chosen by my eldest son Iain. All three boys were given a soft toy each to give to Ishka for Christmas, and they each were told to name them. Ishka chewed and sucked the other two 'cuddlies' to death, and she decided herself to choose 'Chopsticks' as her favourite toy.

I would like to tell you about a game Ishka and I used to play. I thought it might be good practice, because I did not know how bad the eyesight would be for whomever was hopefully going to have her as their guide. If Ishka was out of the room in the house, or out of sight in the garden or on a walk in the woods, I would stand still and close my eyes. I would deliberately have my back from where she might appear. Next, I would put both arms down by my side with palms facing outwards and call her. I would call 'Where's Ishka, Ishka, where's Ishka?' I would then turn around a bit and gesture as to where she might be. She always stopped what she was doing and came within a minute of hearing me. However, it wasn't good enough to just arrive, so I would continue calling her even when she was by my side until she nudged me. Bingo! That was all I wanted, so as a reward we then played with her favourite toy, and I gave her lots of praise. I loved playing that game because it was so special when she made contact with her nose.

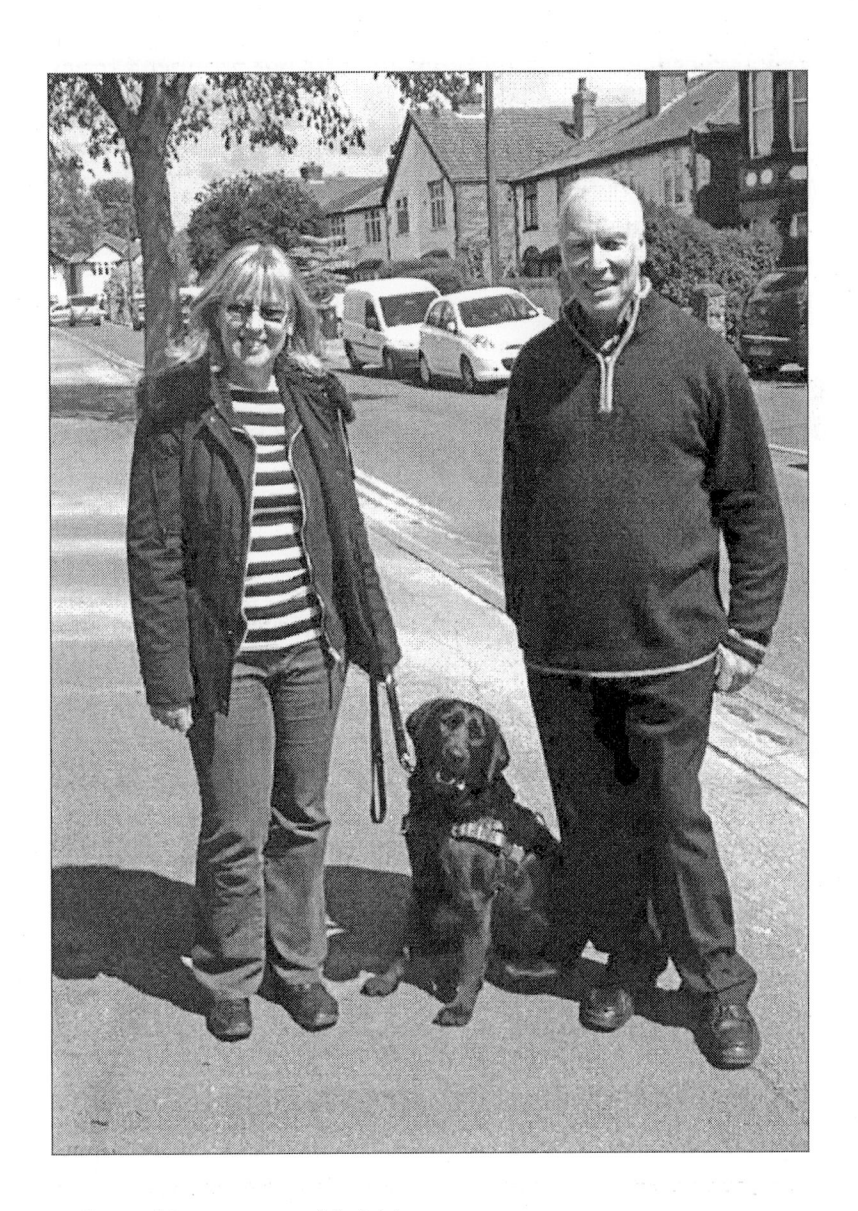

Julie and Lawrence with Ishka.

Ishka went back to 'Guide Dogs' to start her advanced training at Atherton—she returned on Wednesday 7th December 2011. We went on a Shearing's weekend break to Sandown in the Isle of Wight. I had not been to Sandown since I was a child, but thought that it would be a good idea and the perfect distraction for us. On the coach, we found ourselves sitting immediately behind some partially-sighted people. They used a long cane and a most unusual telescope to see certain things more clearly—we were amazed. When we returned home, we were kept busy organising everything for Christmas and the New Year in the Isle of Man.

Lawrence and I met Laraine on our trip down to Nottingham in May 2012 when we saw Ishka for the last time in her advanced stage of training. What an emotional and special day that was. Laraine is a lovely person and so in tune with the dogs. She has a special way that gets results. A letter arrived from 'Guide Dogs' inviting us to a puppy walker's morning at the kennels in Nottingham; where Ishka was based for advanced training. We had no hesitation in accepting the invitation and decided to stay overnight in Nottingham to avoid any travel disruption that might cause delays—we did not want to miss this chance of watching Ishka do some advanced training. We booked at the hotel and took time off to be there. Obviously, this was going to be a very important date for us and I kept wondering what I should wear and what to take—most importantly the camera, of course.

The great day finally came. It was a Wednesday and we had arrived the previous evening which enabled us to find the kennels and then back to the hotel for the night. After breakfast, we set off to the kennels arriving half an hour ahead of schedule and being the first of the visitors to arrive. We were greeted by trainers Laraine and Liz then taken to the comfortable and warm waiting room entertained by Heir Hunters on TV. Other puppy walkers arrived to see their puppies, Ascot and Danny. We chatted over mugs of tea until Liz and Laraine were ready to start the tour of the kennels where the puppies work, eat, sleep and play. Liz and Laraine inform each of us on the progress of their training and also, most importantly, where each dog was going to be living and with whom. Ascot was going to Doncaster with Simon who is a student at Sheffield University, Danny to Sheffield with Kevin and Ishka was being partnered with a lady from Chesterfield. That was the moment that told me that Ishka was going to make the grade—I was elated! I was on cloud nine on hearing the news. It was the start of one of the happiest days of my life.

We were then taken outside to see the obstacle course and as we watched hidden behind bushes so we did not distract the dogs, we were given a running commentary by Liz as each dog performed with Laraine. Ishka was saved until last; she looked so grown up and happy. It had been five months since we said our goodbyes. A feeling of immense pride came over us. We watched her having a great time avoiding the obstacles, but you could see her thinking and working out the best route to get Laraine through safely.

After that had finished we were told that we were going into town to witness the puppies in a real situation amongst the public. We all got into our cars and followed convoy style un-

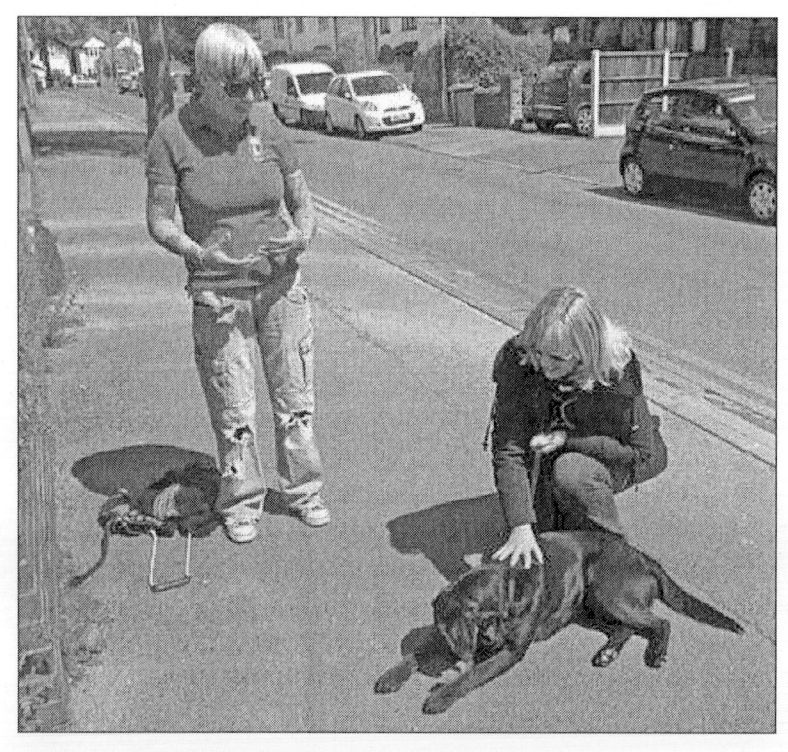

Julie saying goodbye to Ishka

til we reached a car park. Again we were asked to go and enjoy a coffee or walk around the shops until it was our turn to watch Ishka in a real life situation and again, the best was saved to the last (I am biased!), so we went for a coffee. Now, it was Ishka's turn—Laraine put the harness on and with a few words from Laraine she set off with confident strides, then she suddenly starts to slow down and almost stops—oh no, what's going on, then we noticed that a cat was lurking between vehicles along the route. Ishka had spotted the cat and just needed to be sure it was safe to continue. With a reassuring look at her handler she continued—she continued avoiding pedestrians zigzagging along. Even when confronted suddenly by a small tethered dog that leapt out barking from behind an advertising board. Ishka negotiated steps and ramps without hesitation.

The working demonstration completed, it was now our time to share a few precious moments with Ishka again, knowing that this would be the last time. No sadness here, just elation after witnessing how well she had behaved. We spent the rest of the day in the city centre.

The next step in this amazing story was receiving an official communication from Guide Dogs Association that Ishka had qualified as a guide dog then to see it in print in the *Guide Dogs Forward* magazine for autumn 2012: Jean Reid & Ishka from Chesterfield, Anne Julie Macleod from Douglas, and Lyn Shaw from Redditch.

APPENDIX TWO

Block Manual

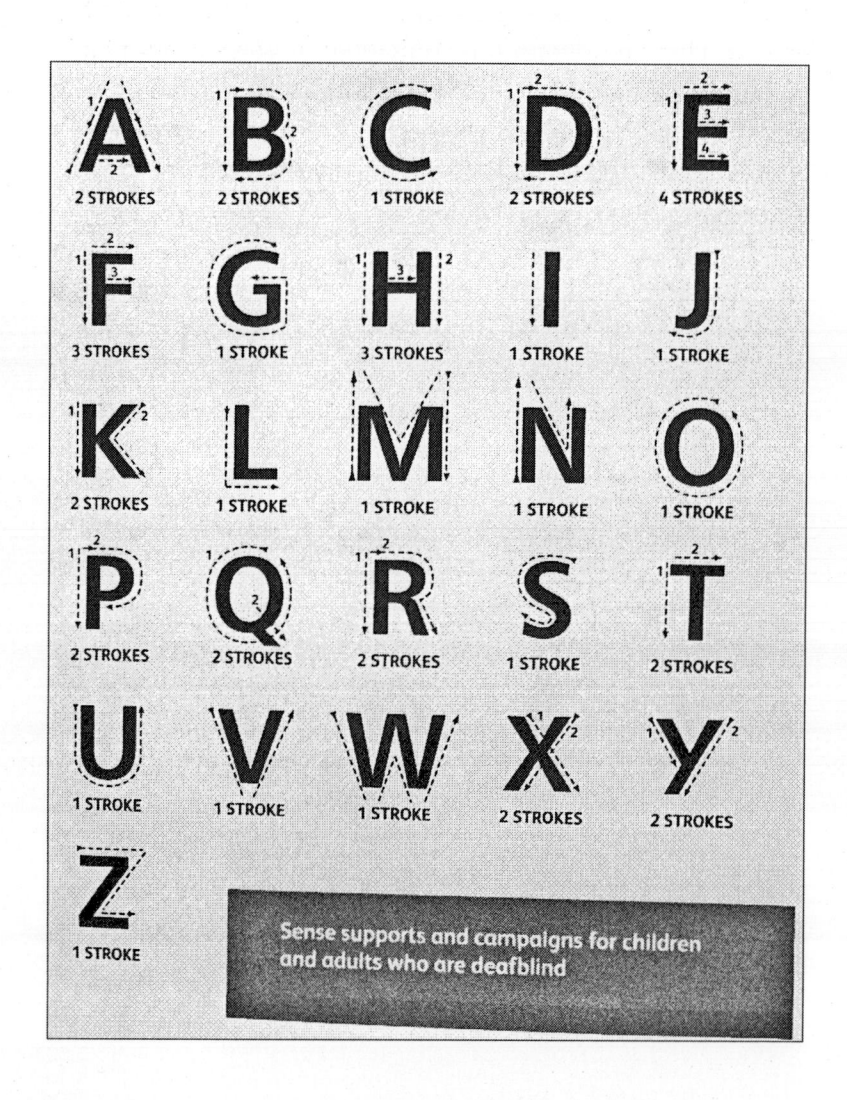

This is a simple system used by some deaf/blind people. With your forefinger draw the clear shape of capital letters on the palm of the deaf/blind person's hand. Use the whole palm for each letter—keeping them large and clear. Place one letter over the top of the last—do not attempt to write across the palm as you would on a sheet of paper and keep your pen in your pocket! Pause slightly at the end of each word making sure the person is able to follow what you are saying. Letters should generally be drawn from left to right and from top to bottom. Letters M, N and W should be drawn keeping the finger on the palm and not in separate strokes. Numbers can alternatively be drawn as figures. Do not use the Continental (7) as this is easily confused as (2).

The image opposite is reproduced courtesy of Sense, the organisation for deafblind people.

APPENDIX THREE

The Deaf/blind Alphabet Manual

The Deaf/blind Manual is the best way to communicate with someone who is Deaf/blind. You can learn it quickly and here's how you do it: Stick out your index finger (that's the long one next to your thumb) on your right hand. fold your other fingers out of the way. Think of this finger as your pen. You are going to use it to write—not on paper, but on your deaf/blind friend's left hand which they will hold out for you. First learn the vowels. They are easy. Just remember the order A, E, I, O, U.

✦ For A, touch the tip of your friend's thumb.

✦ For E, touch the tip of the index finger.

✦ For I, touch the middle finger.

✦ For O, touch the ring finger.

✦ For U, touch the little finger.

And now for the complete alphabet.

✦ For A, touch the tip of your friend's thumb.

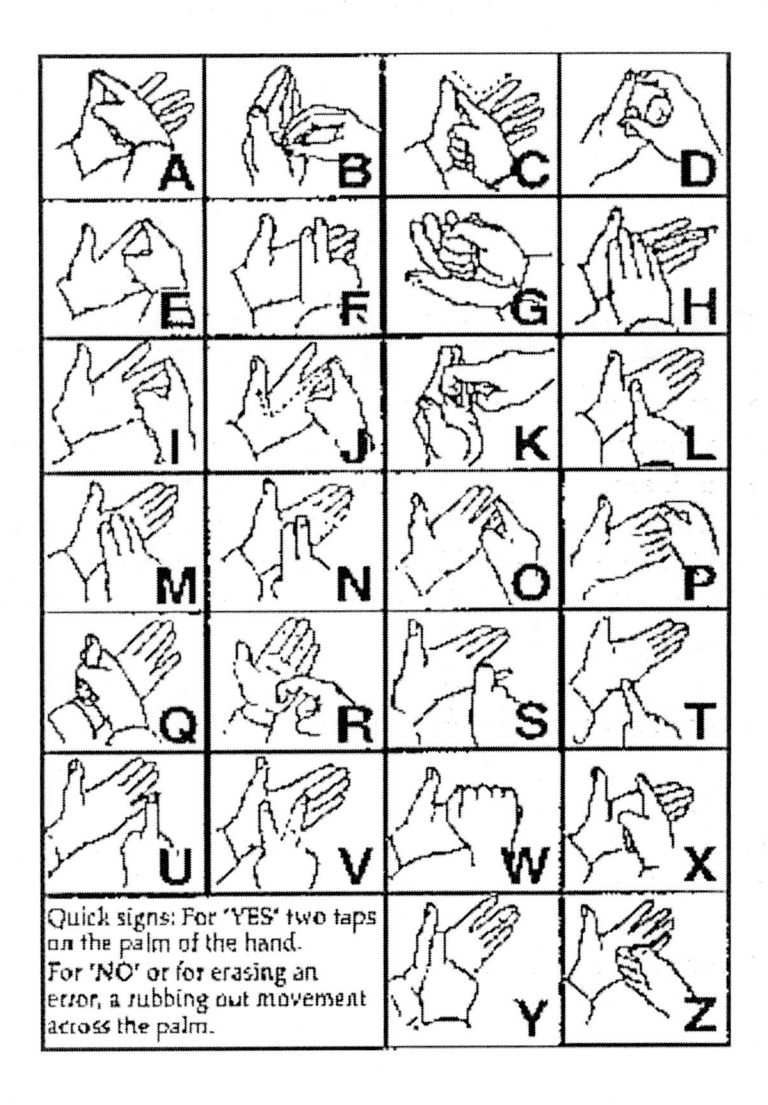

Quick signs: For 'YES' two taps on the palm of the hand.
For 'NO' or for erasing an error, a rubbing out movement across the palm.

Courtesy of James Gallagher

✦ For B, bunch the tips of your fingers and place them on your friend's palm.

✦ For C, use your index finger to make a circular movement that starts on the inside of your friend's thumb and ends at the top of their index finger.

✦ For D, form a D shape using your thumb and index finger and placing it on your friend's index finger.

✦ For E, touch the tip of your friend's index finger.

✦ For F, form an F shape using your first two fingers together, place across your friend's index finger.

✦ For G, clench your fist and place it on your friend's palm, little finger downside.

✦ For H, lay your open hand across your friend's palm and move it over the fingers and off the hand.

✦ For I, touch the tip of your friend's middle finger.

✦ For J, touch the tip of your friend's middle finger and draw your finger down to the palm and up the thumb. (Think of this as the letter I with a tail).

✦ For K, bend your index finger and lay the top half of it against your friend's index finger.

✦ For L, just lay your index finger across your friend's palm.

- For M, lay your first three fingers across your friend's palm.

- For N, lay your first two fingers across your friend's palm.

- For O, touch the tip of your friend's ring finger.

- For P, hold the tip of your friend's index finger between your finger and thumb.

- For Q, completely circle the base of your friend's thumb with your thumb and index finger.

- For R, bend your index finger and lay it across your friend's palm.

- For S, grasp your friend's little finger with your index finger.

- For T, touch the edge of your friend's palm, at the side away from the thumb.

- For U, touch the tip of your friend's little finger.

- For V, make a V shape with your first two fingers and lay it on your friend's palm.

- For W, grasp the upper edge of your friend's fingers, bending your fingers around them.

- For X, make a cross by laying your index finger over the top of your friend's index finger.

✦ For Y, place your index finger in the joint between your friend's thumb and index finger.

✦ For Z, either: place your fingertips against your friend's palm. Or place the outer edge of your hand across your friend's palm.

And now two quick signs that come in handy.

✦ For YES, just tap twice on your friend's palm.

✦ For NO, (or cancelling what you just said) do a rubbing out movement on your friend's palm.

Useful addresses

Sense
Address: Sense, 101 Pentonville Road, London N1 9LG.
Tel: 0300 330 9250.
Website: www.sense.org.uk.

Royal National Institute for the Blind
Address: Registered Charity Number 226227, 105 Judd Street, London WC1H 9NE.
Website: www.rnib.org.uk.

Guide Dogs for the Blind Association
Address: Burgfield Common, Reading RG7 3YG.
Tel: 0118 983 5555.
Website: www.guidedogs.org.uk.
Registered Charity No 20961.

British Retinitis Pigmentosa Society
Address: P.O. Box 370, Buckingham, Buckinghamshire MK18 1GZ.
Tel: 0845 123 2354.
Fax: 01280 815 900.
E.mail: helpline@rpfightingblindenss.org.uk.
Website: www.rpfightingblindness.org.uk.

continued over the page...

Fighting Blindness
Address: P.O. Box 370, Buckingham MK18 1GZ.
E Mail: info@fightingblindness.org.uk.

Action on Hearing Loss (the trading name of the Royal National Institute for Deaf People RNID).
Registered Office: Action on Hearing Loss, RNID, 19–23 Featherstone Street, London, EC1Y 8SL.
Website: www.actiononhearingloss.org.uk/about-us.aspx.